Handbook of
Clinical Dental Assisting

Handbook of
Clinical
Dental
Assisting

Gregory M. Schuster, D.D.S.

in Private Practice, Sumner, Washington

Formerly Clinical Instructor, Bates Technical College
Tacoma, Washington

Gregory J. Wetterhus, D.D.S.

in Private Practice, Puyallup, Washington

Formerly Clinical Instructor, Bates Technical College
Tacoma, Washington

Phyllis Dryden, B.A., C.D.A.

Clinical Director, Dental Assisting Program,
Bates Technical College
Tacoma, Washington

617.6
S395

W.B. SAUNDERS COMPANY
A Division of Harcourt Brace & Company
Philadelphia London Toronto Montreal Sydney Tokyo

WITHDRAWN
LIBRARY
MILWAUKEE AREA TECHNICAL COLLEGE
Milwaukee Campus

W. B. SAUNDERS COMPANY

A Division of Harcourt Brace & Company

The Curtis Center
Independence Square West
Philadelphia, Pennsylvania 19106

Library of Congress Cataloging-in-Publication Data

Schuster, Gregory M.
    Handbook of clinical dental assisting / Gregory M. Schuster,
Gregory J. Wetterhus, Phyllis Dryden. — 1st ed.
      p. cm.
    Includes bibliographical references and index.
    ISBN 0–7216–4536–4
    1. Dental assistants. 2. Dentistry. I. Wetterhus, Gregory J.
II. Dryden, Phyllis. III. Title.
    [DNLM: 1. Dental Assistants. 2. Dental Care. 3. Dental
Assistants examination questions. 4. Dental Care examination
questions. WU 90 S395h 1999]
    RK60.5.S345 1999
    617.6—dc21
    DNLM/DC   98–24847

HANDBOOK OF CLINICAL DENTAL ASSISTING   ISBN 0-7216-4536-4

Last digit is the print number: 9   8   7   6   5   4   3   2   1

Preface

Two objectives the authors endeavor to achieve for the learning dental assistant are organization and preparation for clinical procedures. Once accomplished, the dental assistant can begin learning the art of anticipation, for at this level the dental assistant and dentist together achieve teamwork in the highest sense and the rewards that follow.

In Chapter 1, we outline many common clinical procedures, ranging from operatory preparation and tray setups to breakdown and disinfection of the operatory. This material forms the majority of the handbook and is intended to accomplish the two objectives described above. Under the "Barriers" and "Finish" headings, please refer to "Sterilization and Infection Control" in Chapter 2 for a discussion on the "Spray-Wipe-Spray" technique and other infection control procedures. We minimize the core number of tray setups necessary for inventory purposes and add specific items for various procedures; we recommend a discussion with the instructor/doctor regarding any postoperative instructions prior to addressing the patient.

Chapter 2 highlights many of the duties of dental assistants. Many states now allow expanded duties for dental assistants, including the coronal polish, fluoride application, occlusal sealant application, shade matching, and placement of gingival retraction cord, which provide more opportunity for responsibility and career fulfillment. We strongly urge the users of this handbook to check current state laws and regulations regarding dental practice prior to employing these procedures. New materials and technology are being developed and improved daily, including laser and air-abrasion technology and a host of dentin bonding agents and composite materials such as compomers and flowable composites. We have tried to incorporate familiar, universal standards for materials and techniques in these procedures that can be modified to suit a large audience.

Chart forms and chart entries are discussed in detail in Chapter 3, along with various referral forms for dental specialists and laboratory technicians. Here, we use specific forms and examples that will vary from institution to institution and from private practice to private practice. Behavioral objectives and rationale are provided for several important operative procedures in Chapter 4. We have also included three Appendixes containing answers to study questions, commonly used abbreviations, and evaluation forms to monitor students' progress.

When this material is used, we find the student to be prepared, organized, and better able to participate actively in operative procedures, while the doctor/instructor has more time for instruction and guidance. It is not our intention to provide extensive background material. We assume that students who use this handbook have already completed preclinical procedures and concepts from a comprehensive textbook such as Torres and Ehrlich's *Modern Dental Assisting* (5th edition). Our purpose, rather, is to augment such a textbook with a practical format for success in clinical situations.

The authors would like to welcome to the dental profession all those who use this handbook. It is our goal that the accomplished dental assistant will have many enjoyable and rewarding years in the field.

Gregory M. Schuster, D.D.S.
Gregory J. Wetterhus, D.D.S.
Phyllis Dryden, B.A., C.D.A.

Acknowledgments

The authors wish to acknowledge, first, their loving spouses and families, without whose constant support and patience this effort would not have been possible. Secondly, we thank Selma Kaszczuk, Senior Editor, Health Related Professions, W. B. Saunders; and Rachael Kelly, Assistant Developmental Editor, Health Related Professions, W. B. Saunders, for the opportunity and continued confidence in this, our first publication.

We also thank Jim Clark, Staff Photographer, University of Washington School of Dentistry, Department of Orthodontics, for his expertise in the layout and development of the photographs used throughout the text.

Finally, we give our thanks to the W. B. Saunders staff for the professional support we received during the production of this work: Shirley Kuhn, Acquisitions Editor; Joan Sinclair, Production Manager; and Mary McDonald, Senior Production Editor, P. M. Gordon Associates, Inc.

Contents

Chapter One
Assisting Clinical Procedures 1

Handbook of
Clinical Dental Assisting

Assisting Clinical Procedures

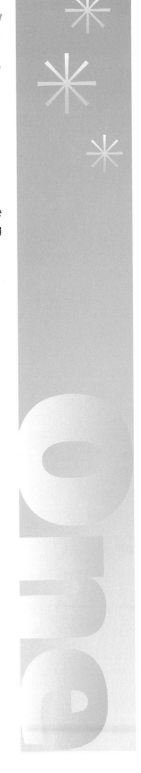

Objectives

After completing this chapter, the dental assistant will be familiar with the sequence of clinical operations and able to prepare the operatory properly for the following clinical procedures:

Adult Initial Examination

Child Initial Examination

Emergency Examination

Amalgam Procedure

Composite Procedure

Crown and Bridge Preparation Procedure

Temporary Crown Fabrication Procedure

Crown and Bridge Seating Procedure

Root Canal Open and Broach/Instrumentation Procedure

Root Canal Obturation Procedure

Post Buildup Procedure

Cast Post and Core Procedure

Removable Partial Dentures (Preparation and Impression)

Removable Partial Dentures (Framework Try-In)

Removable Partial Dentures (Delivery and Postop)

Complete Dentures (Final Impressions)

Complete Dentures (Maxillary–Mandibular Relations)

Complete Dentures (Clinical Wax Try-In)

Complete Dentures (Delivery and Postop)

ERA Attachment Fabrication Procedure

Periodontal Scaling and Polish

Oral Surgery/Extractions

Incision and Drain Procedure

Sealant Application Procedure

Vital Bleaching Tray Fabrication Procedure

Vital Bleaching Tray Delivery Procedure

Occlusal Splint Records Procedure

Occlusal Splint Fabrication Procedure

Occlusal Splint Reline and Delivery Procedure

Occlusal Splint Adjustment Procedure

The new patient examination is the critical first step in developing a long-lasting relationship among the doctor, patient, and dental office staff. Primary objectives for the dental assistant are to

1. welcome the patient and establish rapport
2. record the patient's problems or concerns
3. record all data accurately during the examination, enabling the doctor to establish a working diagnosis and an appropriate plan of care for the patient

The authors suggest recording a facebow transfer and centric relation record to mount accurately the study models taken from the exam on a semiadjustable articulator. The material outlined below will help the dental assistant to enhance the interaction between the patient and the dental team.

Operatory Preparation

Barriers

Prior to seating the patient, the dental assistant will place appropriate infection control barriers in the operatory. These include plastic covering for all surfaces that may become contaminated and that will not be disinfected with an aerosol spray following the procedure. Such surfaces may include

- overhead light handles and light switches
- operatory delivery systems
- plastic tubing for handpieces and suction
- nitrous oxide equipment
- x-ray heads
- doctor and assistant stools
- headrest on the dental chair

Personal protective equipment (eyewear, masks, and gloves) will be available and ready to use during the procedure for both the doctor and the dental assistant. Protective eyewear will also be provided for the patient.

Exam Tray (Fig. 1-1)

- ✓ instruments (mouth mirror, explorer, periodontal probe, cotton pliers, etc.)
- ✓ 2×2s
- ✓ cotton rolls
- ✓ high-volume evacuator
- ✓ saliva ejector
- ✓ air-water tip
- ✓ articulating paper on forceps
- ✓ blood pressure equipment
- ✓ stock metal trays and premeasured alginate and water
- ✓ spatula and bowl
- ✓ bite registration material
- ✓ facebow

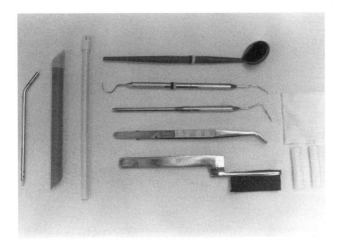

Figure 1-1. Standard tray setup for the adult new patient examination. Tray setup includes, from left to right: air-water tip, high-volume evacuator (HVE), saliva ejector, mouth mirror, explorer, periodontal probe, cotton pliers, articulating paper on forceps, gauze 2×2s, and cotton rolls.

Seating Patient

The dental assistant:

* ✳ Greets the patient and places the bib
* ✳ Takes blood pressure and records in the patient chart
* ✳ Reviews the health history with the patient; identifies any allergies (especially latex, medications) and all medications (with dosages) the patient is currently taking
* ✳ Takes the appropriate radiographs as instructed by the doctor (bitewings, periapicals, full mouth series, and/or panoramic)
* ✳ Takes the appropriate alginate impressions and facebow transfer as instructed by the doctor

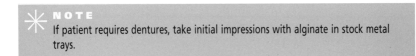

> ✳ **NOTE**
> If patient requires dentures, take initial impressions with alginate in stock metal trays.

* ✳ Charts existing restorations on Examination Form
* ✳ Has notepad ready to write notes

Upon completion of the above steps, the dental assistant summons the doctor to begin the exam.

Examination

The dental assistant:

* Introduces the doctor to the patient
* Has the mouth mirror, explorer, and Examination Form ready
* Records intraoral and radiographic findings and helps to formulate treatment as instructed by the doctor
* Assists the doctor in obtaining a centric relation record
* Asks the doctor for the next appointment
* Removes the bib and walks the patient to the front desk

The dental assistant will now remove all the plastic barriers in the operatory, replace them with new ones, and spray all contaminated surfaces with an Occupational Safety and Health Administration (OSHA)-approved disinfectant to get the operatory ready for the next patient.

> **NOTE**
> The authors suggest that users of this text review their current state infection control regulations and modify these procedures if necessary.

Child Initial Examination

The child initial examination is as critical as the adult new patient examination in developing a long-lasting relationship among the doctor, child and parents, and dental office staff. Primary objectives for the dental assistant are to

1. welcome and help make the child feel comfortable
2. record the patient's problems or concerns
3. accurately record all data during the examination, enabling the doctor to establish a working diagnosis and an appropriate plan of care for the child

The material outlined below will help the dental assistant to enhance the interaction between the child and the dental team.

Operatory Preparation

Barriers

Prior to seating the patient, the dental assistant will place appropriate infection control barriers in the operatory. These include plastic covering for all surfaces that may become contaminated and that will not be disinfected with an aerosol spray following the procedure. Such surfaces may include

- overhead light handles and light switches
- operatory delivery systems
- plastic tubing for handpieces and suction
- nitrous oxide equipment
- x-ray heads
- doctor and assistant stools
- headrest on the dental chair

Personal protective equipment (eyewear, masks, and gloves) will be available and ready to use during the procedure for both the doctor and the dental assistant. Protective eyewear will also be provided for the patient.

Exam Tray (Fig. 1-2)

✓ instruments (mouth mirror, explorer, cotton pliers, etc.)
✓ 2×2s
✓ cotton rolls
✓ high-volume evacuator
✓ saliva ejector
✓ air-water tip

Seating Patient

The dental assistant:

* Walks out to the waiting room, introduces self to both the parent and the child, and notes in the chart the child's preferred name

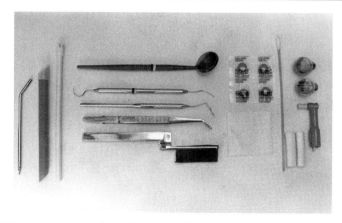

Figure 1-2. Standard tray setup for child new patient examination and recall appointments. Note the disclosing tablets to be used during oral hygiene instruction.

✳ Reviews the health history with the parent; identifies any allergies (especially latex, medications) and all medications (with dosages) the child is currently taking
✳ Asks the parent if there are any special concerns regarding the child prior to the examination
✳ Lets the parent know that he or she will be coming back to the operatory at the end of the appointment and approximately how long the appointment will last
✳ Seats the child and places the bib
✳ Takes the appropriate radiographs as instructed by the doctor (bitewings, occlusals, panoramic)
✳ Charts existing restorations on the Examination Form
✳ Has notepad ready to write notes

Examination

The dental assistant:

✳ Discloses the child and begins oral hygiene instruction
✳ Completes the coronal polish and flosses all teeth
✳ Administers topical fluoride treatment
✳ Introduces the child to the doctor

The doctor now examines the teeth and gums, and performs a head and neck examination.

Examination Summary and Finish

The doctor:

- ✳ Has the dental assistant bring the parent to the operatory
- ✳ Discusses the diseases of the mouth with the parent
- ✳ Reviews findings of decay and defective fillings
- ✳ Reviews the child's oral hygiene
- ✳ Advises the parent of appropriate referrals (e.g., orthodontist) and has the parent sign the consent form
- ✳ Asks the parent if there are any questions

The dental assistant:

- ✳ Asks the doctor for the next appointment
- ✳ Removes the bib and walks the child and parent to the front desk

The dental assistant will now remove all the plastic barriers in the operatory, replace them with new ones, and spray all contaminated surfaces with an OSHA-approved disinfectant to get the operatory ready for the next patient.

NOTE
The authors suggest that users of this text review their current state infection control regulations and modify these procedures if necessary.

When working with the patient experiencing pain, either an established or a new patient, it is important to exercise caution when using any instruments, air, water, or suction. Every effort should be made to help comfort the patient.

Operatory Preparation

Barriers

Prior to seating the patient, the dental assistant will place appropriate infection control barriers in the operatory. These include plastic covering for all surfaces that may become contaminated and that will not be disinfected with an aerosol spray following the procedure. Such surfaces may include

- overhead light handles and light switches
- operatory delivery systems
- plastic tubing for handpieces and suction
- nitrous oxide equipment
- x-ray heads
- doctor and assistant stools
- headrest on the dental chair

Personal protective equipment (eyewear, masks, and gloves) will be available and ready to use during the procedure for both the doctor and the dental assistant. Protective eyewear will also be provided for the patient.

Exam Tray (Fig. 1-3)

- ✓ instruments (mouth mirror, explorer, periodontal probe, cotton pliers, etc.)
- ✓ 2×2s
- ✓ cotton rolls
- ✓ "Tooth Slooth"
- ✓ high-volume evacuator
- ✓ saliva ejector
- ✓ air-water tip
- ✓ articulating paper on forceps
- ✓ cold test equipment
- ✓ heat test equipment
- ✓ electric pulp tester

Seating Patient

The dental assistant:

* Greets the patient and places the bib
* Reviews the health history with the patient; identifies any allergies (especially latex, medications) and all medications (with dosages) the patient is currently taking

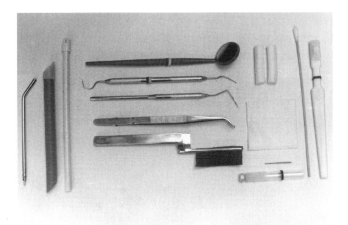

Figure 1-3. Standard tray setup for an emergency examination. Note the ice and gutta percha cones for cold and heat pulp testing equipment and the "Tooth Slooth."

✳ Takes periapical radiograph of the painful area
✳ Has a notepad ready to write notes
✳ Summons the doctor to begin the examination

Examination

The dental assistant:

✳ Introduces the patient (if a new patient) to the doctor
✳ Has mouth mirror, explorer, and treatment plan ready

The doctor may perform the following tests:

✳ Percussion test
✳ Cold test
✳ Use "Tooth Slooth" or wet cotton roll for cracked tooth syndrome
✳ Check occlusion
✳ Probe pocket depths
✳ Check mobility
✳ Heat test

After radiographic analysis, the doctor will discuss the treatment options with the patient (root canal treatment, extraction, referral, prescriptions, no treatment, etc.). The dental assistant now informs the doctor if enough time is available to perform the recommended treatment. If there is not enough time, the patient is given an appointment for the next available time. Following the procedure, the bib is removed and the patient is brought to the front desk.

The dental assistant will now remove all the plastic barriers in the operatory, replace them with new ones, and spray all contaminated surfaces with an OSHA-approved disinfectant to get the operatory ready for the next patient.

> ✳ **N O T E**
> The authors suggest that users of this text review their current state infection control regulations and modify these procedures if necessary.

Amalgam Procedure

Operatory Preparation

Barriers

Prior to seating the patient, the dental assistant will place appropriate infection control barriers in the operatory. These include plastic covering for all surfaces that may become contaminated and that will not be disinfected with an aerosol spray following the procedure. Such surfaces may include

- overhead light handles and light switches
- operatory delivery systems
- plastic tubing for handpieces and suction
- nitrous oxide equipment
- x-ray heads
- doctor and assistant stools
- headrest on the dental chair

Personal protective equipment (eyewear, masks, and gloves) will be available and ready to use during the procedure for both the doctor and the dental assistant. Protective eyewear will also be provided for the patient.

Amalgam Tray (Fig. 1-4A,B)

- ✓ instruments (mouth mirror, explorer, periodontal probe, cotton pliers, spoon excavator)
- ✓ amalgam carriers and condensers
- ✓ amalgam carvers [e.g., Walls, Hollenbeck, Cleoid-Discoid]
- ✓ 2×2s
- ✓ cotton rolls
- ✓ high-volume evacuator
- ✓ saliva ejector
- ✓ air-water tip
- ✓ articulating paper on forceps
- ✓ cotton tip with topical
- ✓ anesthetic syringe
- ✓ two Carpules of anesthetic
- ✓ dental dam setup and clamps
- ✓ floss
- ✓ wedges
- ✓ matrix bands

After tray setup is complete, the dental assistant will set up the following:

* Handpieces: high-speed with fissure bur (e.g., #56) prerun with water and fiberoptics on
  slow-speed with round bur (e.g., #6)
* Anesthetic: 30-gauge needle for maxillary and children
  27- or 30-gauge needle for mandibular, depending on doctor's preference
* Tofflemire matrix bands and retainers

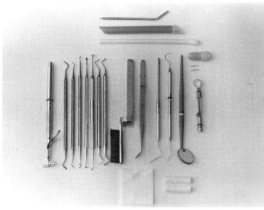
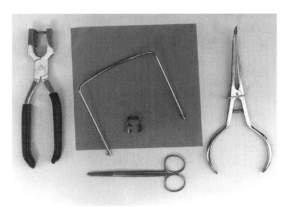

A

B

Figure 1-4. (**A**) Standard tray setup for amalgam procedure, including the Tofflemire matrix and retainer. Note the amalgam condensers and carving instruments that distinguish this tray from other restorative tray setups. (**B**) Materials for dental dam application for amalgam, composite, crown and bridge, and endodontic procedures.

✳ Dental dam and appropriate clamp
✳ Bitewing or periapical radiographs in viewbox

Seating Patient

The dental assistant:

✳ Greets the patient, places the bib, and discusses the appointment with the patient
✳ Asks the patient if there are any changes in his or her health history
✳ Makes chart entries and has notepad ready to write notes
✳ Places topical in correct area and summons the doctor

Examination

The dental assistant:

✳ Has mouth mirror, explorer, and treatment plan ready
✳ Passes anesthetic syringe to the doctor

Isolation

The dental assistant:

✳ Places the dental dam or cotton rolls at the doctor's request.

Preparation

The doctor prepares the tooth (teeth).
The dental assistant places the matrix band(s) and wedge(s).
Optional items that the doctor may need are liners, desensitizers, pins, etc.

Fill

The doctor:

* ✳ Fills the tooth (teeth), removes the wedges and matrix, carves the filling, and removes the dental dam

The dental assistant:

* ✳ Rinses the patient

Finish

The doctor:

* ✳ Clears contact with floss
* ✳ Checks the occlusion with 2×2s and articulating paper

The dental assistant:

* ✳ Provides postoperative instructions as directed by the doctor
* ✳ Finishes the chart entry and asks the doctor for the next appointment
* ✳ Removes the bib and walks the patient to the front desk

The dental assistant will now remove all the plastic barriers in the operatory, replace them with new ones, and spray all contaminated surfaces with an OSHA-approved disinfectant to get the operatory ready for the next patient.

NOTE
The authors suggest that users of this text review their current state infection control regulations and modify these procedures if necessary.

Composite Procedure

Operatory Preparation

Barriers

Prior to seating the patient, the dental assistant will place appropriate infection control barriers in the operatory. These include plastic covering for all surfaces that may become contaminated and that will not be disinfected with an aerosol spray following the procedure. Such surfaces may include

- overhead light handles and light switches
- operatory delivery systems
- plastic tubing for handpieces and suction
- nitrous oxide equipment
- x-ray heads
- doctor and assistant stools
- headrest on the dental chair

Personal protective equipment (eyewear, masks, and gloves) will be available and ready to use during the procedure for both the doctor and the dental assistant. Protective eyewear will also be provided for the patient.

Composite Tray (Fig. 1-5)

- ✓ instruments (mouth mirror, explorer, periodontal probe, cotton pliers, spoon excavator, plastic instrument, composite carvers)
- ✓ 2×2s
- ✓ cotton rolls
- ✓ high-volume evacuator
- ✓ saliva ejector
- ✓ air-water tip
- ✓ articulating paper on forceps
- ✓ cotton tip with topical
- ✓ anesthetic syringe
- ✓ two Carpules of anesthetic
- ✓ dental dam setup and clamps
- ✓ floss
- ✓ wedges
- ✓ clear matrix bands

After tray setup is complete, the dental assistant will set up the following:

* Handpieces: high-speed with fissure bur (e.g., #56 or #330) prerun with water and fiberoptics on
slow-speed with round bur (e.g., #2 or #4), and mandrel ready for finishing discs
* Anesthetic: 30-gauge needle for maxillary and children
27- or 30-gauge needle for mandibular, depending on doctor's preference

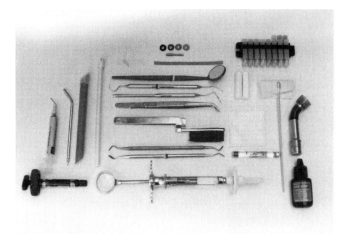

Figure 1-5. Standard tray setup for composite procedure. Note that the etchant, primer and adhesive, composite, and light curing unit may be placed on supplemental trays and/or tubs that can be accessed during the procedure.

* Bi-Tine rings or similar bands for posterior composites only
* Dental dam and appropriate clamp
* Bitewing or periapical radiographs in viewbox
* Composite light-curing unit
* Composite material(s) including liners and shade guide
* Etchant, primer, and bonding resin
* Benda brushes, finishing strips, and discs

Seating Patient

The dental assistant:

* Greets the patient, places the bib, and discusses the appointment with the patient
* Asks the patient if there are any changes in his or her health history
* Chooses the shade, records it in the chart, and confirms it with the doctor
* Makes chart entries and has notepad ready to write notes
* Places topical in the correct area and summons the doctor

Examination

The dental assistant:

* Has mouth mirror, explorer, and treatment plan ready
* Passes anesthetic syringe to the doctor

Isolation

The dental assistant:

* Places the dental dam or cotton rolls at the doctor's request
* Has etchant, primer, adhesive, and composite ready

Preparation and Fill

The doctor prepares the tooth (teeth).

The dental assistant:

* Acid etches the tooth (teeth) for 30 seconds, rinses, and dries
* Places the matrix band(s) and wedge(s)
* Applies primer for 30 seconds and dries
* Applies bonding resin and light cures for 20 seconds

After the doctor applies the composite material, the dental assistant light cures it for 40 seconds on all sides.

> **NOTE**
> The above times for etching, curing, and so on are only examples. The authors recommend that users of this text follow the specific instructions of the manufacturer for each product.

Finish

The dental assistant:

* Removes the wedges, matrix, and dental dam

The doctor:

* Removes excess composite material with finishing burs, discs, and finishing strips
* Checks contact areas with floss

The dental assistant:

* Rinses the patient
* Provides postoperative instructions as directed by the doctor
* Finishes the chart entry while the doctor checks the occlusion with

2×2s and articulating paper, and asks the doctor for the next appointment

✳ Removes the bib and walks the patient to the front desk

The dental assistant will now remove all the plastic barriers in the operatory, replace them with new ones, and spray all contaminated surfaces with an OSHA-approved disinfectant to get the operatory ready for the next patient.

> ✳ **N O T E**
> The authors suggest that users of this text review their current state infection control regulations and modify these procedures if necessary.

Crown and Bridge Preparation Procedure

A wide variety of materials and techniques may be used during a crown or bridge preparation procedure. The authors utilize a two-layer retraction cord technique for improved hemostasis and retraction, full-arch custom acrylic impression trays, polyvinylsiloxane final impression material, a full-arch opposing model, and custom acrylic temporaries. Modifications of this procedure may be necessary, depending on the materials and techniques used in your office. Consult with the doctor prior to the procedure.

Operatory Preparation

Barriers

Prior to seating the patient, the dental assistant will place appropriate infection control barriers in the operatory. These include plastic covering for all surfaces that may become contaminated and that will not be disinfected with an aerosol spray following the procedure. Such surfaces may include

- overhead light handles and light switches
- operatory delivery systems
- plastic tubing for handpieces and suction
- nitrous oxide equipment
- x-ray heads
- doctor and assistant stools
- headrest on the dental chair

Personal protective equipment (eyewear, masks, and gloves) will be available and ready to use during the procedure for both the doctor and the dental assistant. Protective eyewear will also be provided for the patient.

Crown and Bridge Tray (Fig. 1-6)

- ✓ instruments (mouth mirror, explorer, periodontal probe, cotton pliers, spoon excavator, retraction cord placing instruments, plastic instrument, hemostats)
- ✓ 2×2s
- ✓ cotton rolls
- ✓ high-volume evacuator
- ✓ saliva ejector
- ✓ air-water tip
- ✓ articulating paper on forceps
- ✓ cotton tip with topical anesthetic syringe
- ✓ two Carpules of anesthetic
- ✓ dental dam setup and clamps
- ✓ Svedopter
- ✓ floss

After tray setup is complete, the dental assistant will set up the following:

* Handpieces: high-speed with fissure or diamond bur prerun with water and fiberoptics on

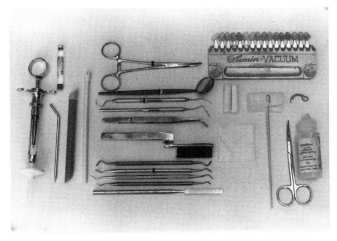

Figure 1-6. Standard tray setup for a crown and bridge preparation procedure. Note the retraction cord and hemostatic agent available.

        slow-speed with round bur (e.g., #2 or #4) and straight nose cone with acrylic bur ready

✳ Anesthetic: 30-gauge needle for maxillary and children

        27- or 30-gauge needle for mandibular, depending on doctor's preference

✳ Precut dental dam and appropriate clamp

✳ Bitewing or periapical radiographs in viewbox

✳ Dappen dish with hemostatic agent

✳ Precut retraction cord of appropriate size

✳ Final impression material and impression syringe

✳ Custom or perforated acrylic trays and tray adhesive

✳ Premeasured alginate and water, spatula and bowl, and stock metal tray for opposing impression

✳ Bite registration material

✳ Clear wax to check occlusion

✳ Dappen dish with acrylic

✳ Vacuform shell, aluminum, polycarbonate, etc., for temporary crown

✳ Temporary cement on pad with spatula

✳ Lab prescription forms and shade guide

Seating Patient

The dental assistant:

✳ Greets the patient, places the bib, and discusses the appointment with the patient

✳ Asks the patient if there are any changes in his or her health history
✳ Chooses the shade, records it on the lab prescription form and in the chart, and later confirms it with the doctor
✳ Tries in impression trays for final impression and opposing model to check fit
✳ Makes chart entries and has notepad ready to write notes
✳ Places topical in correct area and summons the doctor

Examination

The dental assistant:

✳ Has mouth mirror, explorer, and treatment plan ready
✳ Passes anesthetic syringe to the doctor

Isolation

The dental assistant:

✳ Places dental dam, Svedopter, or cotton rolls at doctor's request

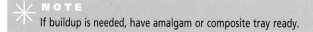

✳ **NOTE**
If buildup is needed, have amalgam or composite tray ready.

Preparation

The doctor prepares the tooth (teeth).

The dental assistant:

✳ Places the retraction cord under the doctor's supervision
✳ Takes the opposing arch impression with alginate
✳ Removes the dental dam

The doctor takes the final impression and bite registration.
The dental assistant fabricates the temporary crown (see the section "Temporary Crown Fabrication Procedure" for an explanation).

Finish

The dental assistant:

✳ Cements the temporary crown with temporary cement
✳ Removes excess cement and flosses around the temporary crown

✳ Rinses the patient and provides postoperative instructions as directed by the doctor
✳ Finishes the chart entries and lab prescription forms
✳ Removes the bib and walks the patient to the front desk

The dental assistant will now remove all the plastic barriers in the operatory, replace them with new ones, and spray all contaminated surfaces with an OSHA-approved disinfectant to get the operatory ready for the next patient.

NOTE
The authors suggest that users of this text review their current state infection control regulations and modify these procedures if necessary.

Temporary Crown Fabrication Procedure

As an adjunct to the crown and bridge procedure, appropriate barriers have already been placed and do not need to be changed at this time since this procedure immediately follows the crown preparation. However, since a vast array of materials and equipment is already present from the previous procedure, it may simplify matters to bring the appropriate materials for the temporary crown procedure to the operatory at this time.

The authors acknowledge that many satisfactory temporary crowns and methods are available, including the custom acrylic crown from a vacuform matrix coping, preformed polycarbonate or metal crowns lined with acrylic, and so on. The method outlined here uses an alginate impression taken from the preprepared tooth and cold cure acrylic.

Operatory Preparation

Crown and Bridge Tray (Fig. 1-7)

✓ instruments (see the section "Crown and Bridge Preparation Procedure")
✓ 2 × 2s
✓ cotton rolls
✓ high-volume evacuator
✓ saliva ejector
✓ air-water tip
✓ articulating paper on forceps
✓ premeasured alginate and water
✓ spatula and bowl
✓ check-bite or full-arch tray for impression or vacuform shell coping or preformed metal/polycarbonate crown

✓ liquid monomer
✓ acrylic powder
✓ metal spatula to mix acrylic and cement
✓ Woodson
✓ hemostats
  scissors
✓ petroleum jelly
✓ temporary cement
✓ slow-speed handpiece with acrylic bur

Fabrication of Temporary Crown

In the following order, the dental assistant will:

1. Take alginate impression of quadrant with check-bite or full-arch tray prior to tooth preparation
2. Try in alginate impression for fit and landmarks after tooth has been prepared

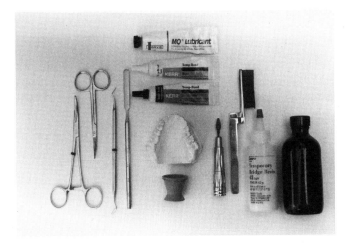

Figure 1-7. Instruments and equipment necessary for the fabrication of a custom acrylic temporary crown, including articulating paper on forceps, vacuform matrix coping, acrylic powder and liquid monomer, mixing spatula, rubber mixing cup, plastic instrument, hemostats, crown and bridge scissors, petroleum jelly, temporary cement, slow-speed handpiece with acrylic bur.

3. Lubricate tooth with petroleum jelly and warm the alginate impression in a warm water bath

4. Mix monomer and acrylic powder in rubber cup until mix begins to form and shine dulls

5. Roll a small amount of the excess acrylic into a ball to evaluate the setting time of the acrylic while the impression is in the mouth

6. Place the mixed acrylic into the area the dental assistant is working on in the alginate impression

7. Carefully place the alginate impression into the patient's mouth, have the patient bite into the check-bite tray or on a cotton roll for full arch impression, and hold for approximately 1 minute or until the ball of excess acrylic begins to warm

8. After 1 minute, have the patient open his or her mouth and remove the alginate impression. The acrylic should have formed to the tooth

9. Mark the margins with a sharp pencil and avoid this line when trimming

10. Remove the acrylic from the tooth, trim the excess acrylic from the crown and gingival margins, try the acrylic temporary on the tooth, have the patient bite softly, and remove the acrylic temporary crown

11. Trim the acrylic temporary crown with a slow-speed handpiece and acrylic bur, contour, and polish with wet pumice and rag wheel on the lathe

Finish

After fabrication of the temporary crown has been completed, the dental assistant:

✳ Checks the occlusion with 2×2s and articulating paper on forceps and makes adjustments as necessary
✳ Cements the acrylic temporary with temporary cement
✳ Provides postoperative instructions as directed by the doctor
✳ Removes excess cement and rinses the patient
✳ Asks the doctor for the next appointment
✳ Removes the bib and walks the patient to the front desk

The dental assistant will now remove all the plastic barriers in the operatory, replace them with new ones, and spray all contaminated surfaces with an OSHA-approved disinfectant to get the operatory ready for the next patient.

NOTE
The authors suggest that users of this text review their current state infection control regulations and modify these procedures if necessary.

Crown and Bridge Seating Procedure

Operatory Preparation

Barriers

Prior to seating the patient, the dental assistant will place appropriate infection control barriers in the operatory. These include plastic covering for all surfaces that may become contaminated and that will not be disinfected with an aerosol spray following the procedure. Such surfaces may include

- overhead light handles and light switches
- operatory delivery systems
- plastic tubing for handpieces and suction
- nitrous oxide equipment
- x-ray heads
- doctor and assistant stools
- headrest on the dental chair

Personal protective equipment (eyewear, masks, and gloves) will be available and ready to use during the procedure for both the doctor and the dental assistant. Protective eyewear will also be provided for the patient.

Crown and Bridge Tray (Fig. 1-8)

- ✓ instruments (mouth mirror, explorer, periodontal probe, cotton pliers, spoon excavator, hemostats)
- ✓ 2×2s
- ✓ cotton rolls
- ✓ high-volume evacuator
- ✓ saliva ejector
- ✓ air-water tip
- ✓ articulating paper on forceps
- ✓ cotton tip with topical
- ✓ anesthetic syringe
- ✓ two Carpules of anesthetic
- ✓ floss
- ✓ permanent crown on model

After tray setup is complete, the dental assistant will set up the following:

* Handpieces: high-speed with green stone prerun with water and fiberoptics on
  slow-speed with straight nose cone and Joe Dandy disc and burlew wheel ready
* Anesthetic: 30-gauge needle for maxillary and children
  27- or 30-gauge needle for mandibular, depending on doctor's preference
* Bitewing or periapical radiographs in viewbox
* Chilled glass slab with zinc phosphate cement or paper pad with glass ionmer cement, etc.; spatula

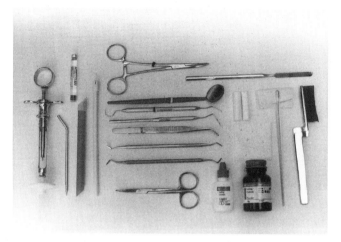

Figure 1-8. Standard tray setup for crown and bridge cementation procedures. Included are a cement spatula, plastic instrument, and crown and bridge scissors.

Seating Patient

The dental assistant:

* Greets the patient, places the bib, and discusses the appointment with the patient
* Asks the patient if there are any changes in his or her health history
* Asks the patient if the tooth has been sensitive
    If "yes," summons the doctor to give anesthetic and places topical in the correct location
    If "no," attempts to remove the temporary; if it does not move or if the patient experiences pain, summons the doctor to give anesthetic and places topical in the correct location

Examination

The dental assistant:

* Has mouth mirror, explorer, and permanent crown on die or model ready
* Passes anesthetic syringe to the doctor if needed

Isolation

The dental assistant:

* Removes the temporary cement from the tooth with cotton pellet
* Places cotton rolls

Seat

The doctor:

* ✳ Evaluates the fit of the crown or bridge and adjusts the shade and contour
* ✳ Checks the interproximal contacts with floss and adjusts
* ✳ Evaluates the margins with the explorer
* ✳ Checks the occlusion with 2×2s and articulating paper on forceps
* ✳ Polishes the crown or bridge
* ✳ Cements the crown or bridge with permanent cement

Finish

The dental assistant:

* ✳ Removes excess cement from the tooth using an explorer and floss
* ✳ Rinses the patient and provides postoperative instructions as directed by the doctor
* ✳ Finishes the chart entry and asks the doctor for the next appointment
* ✳ Removes the bib and walks the patient to the front desk

The dental assistant will now remove all the plastic barriers in the operatory, replace them with new ones, and spray all contaminated surfaces with an OSHA-approved disinfectant to get the operatory ready for the next patient.

NOTE
The authors suggest that users of this text review their current state infection control regulations and modify these procedures if necessary.

A wide variety of materials and techniques may be used during endodontic procedures. Following is an outline of the root canal procedures for instrumentation and obturation consistent with a vertically compacted, warm gutta percha technique. Prior to using these procedures, consult with the doctor for appropriate instruments and materials.

Operatory Preparation

Barriers

Prior to seating the patient, the dental assistant will place appropriate infection control barriers in the operatory. These include plastic covering for all surfaces that may become contaminated and that will not be disinfected with an aerosol spray following the procedure. Such surfaces may include

- overhead light handles and light switches
- operatory delivery systems
- plastic tubing for handpieces and suction
- nitrous oxide equipment
- x-ray heads
- doctor and assistant stools
- headrest on the dental chair

Personal protective equipment (eyewear, masks, and gloves) will be available and ready to use during the procedure for both the doctor and the dental assistant. Protective eyewear will also be provided for the patient.

Endodontic Tray (Fig. 1-9)

- ✓ instruments (mouth mirror, explorer, endodontic explorer, periodontal probe, cotton pliers, spoon excavator, hemostats)
- ✓ 2×2s
- ✓ cotton rolls
- ✓ high-volume evacuator
- ✓ saliva ejector
- ✓ air-water tip
- ✓ articulating paper on forceps
- ✓ cotton tip with topical
- ✓ anesthetic syringe
- ✓ two Carpules of anesthetic
- ✓ floss
- ✓ endodontic ruler

After tray setup is complete, the dental assistant will set up the following:

* Handpieces: high-speed with fissure bur (e.g., #56) prerun with water and fiberoptics on

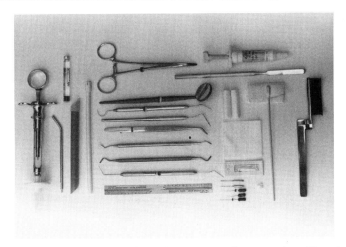

Figure 1-9. Standard tray setup for root canal instrumentation procedure. Note the Gates-Glidden burs, broaches, and files.

                    slow-speed with round bur (e.g., #6) with Gates-Glidden burs and rotary instruments ready

* Anesthetic: 30-gauge needle for maxillary and children

                    27- or 30-gauge needle for mandibular, depending on doctor's preference
* Bitewing or periapical radiographs in viewbox
* Precut dental dam with one hole only and appropriate clamp
* Slip of paper for working lengths and corresponding files
* Sodium hypochlorite, hydrogen peroxide, and irrigating syringe
* Files and reamers (#08–#70) in sponge
* Gates-Glidden burs (#2–#5)
* Broaches, paper points (medium and fine), cotton pellets, medicated cotton pellet, dappen dish, CAVIT, x-ray film, and RC Prep

Seating Patient

The dental assistant:

* Greets the patient, places the bib, and discusses the appointment with the patient
* Asks the patient if there are any changes in his or her health history
* Makes chart entries and has notepad ready to write notes
* Places topical in correct area and summons the doctor

Examination

The dental assistant:

✳ Has mouth mirror, explorer, and treatment plan ready
✳ Passes anesthetic syringe to the doctor

Isolation

The dental assistant:

✳ Places the dental dam (only need one hole)

Preparation

The doctor:

✳ Prepares the access cavity
   1. Flares orifice with Gates-Glidden burs
   2. Broaches pulp tissue and establishes working length

The dental assistant:

✳ Takes periapical working length radiograph
✳ Sets remaining files to working length, as instructed by the doctor

The doctor:

✳ Instruments canal(s) with files and/or rotary instruments

The dental assistant:

✳ Irrigates canal(s) with sodium hypochlorite or hydrogen peroxide, as instructed by the doctor, and dries with paper points when instrumentation is finished
✳ Places cotton pellet with medicated solution of doctor's choice
✳ Places temporary (e.g., CAVIT)

Finish

The dental assistant:

✳ Reviews the procedure and explains postoperative instructions to the patient as directed by the doctor
✳ Gives the patient any prescriptions the doctor has written
✳ Rinses the patient after removal of the dental dam
✳ Checks occlusion with 2×2s and articulating paper on forceps

* Finishes chart entry and asks the doctor for the next appointment
* Removes the bib and walks the patient to the front desk

The dental assistant will now remove all the plastic barriers in the operatory, replace them with new ones, and spray all contaminated surfaces with an OSHA-approved disinfectant to get the operatory ready for the next patient.

NOTE
The authors suggest that users of this text review their current state infection control regulations and modify these procedures if necessary.

Root Canal Obturation Procedure

Operatory Preparation

Barriers

Prior to seating the patient, the dental assistant will place appropriate infection control barriers in the operatory. These include plastic covering for all surfaces that may become contaminated and that will not be disinfected with an aerosol spray following the procedure. Such surfaces may include

- overhead light handles and light switches
- operatory delivery systems
- plastic tubing for handpieces and suction

- nitrous oxide equipment
- x-ray heads
- doctor and assistant stools
- headrest on the dental chair

Personal protective equipment (eyewear, masks, and gloves) will be available and ready to use during the procedure for both the doctor and the dental assistant. Protective eyewear will also be provided for the patient.

Endodontic Tray (Fig. 1-10)

- ✓ instruments (mouth mirror, explorer, endodontic explorer, periodontal probe, cotton pliers, spoon excavator, hemostats)
- ✓ 2×2s
- ✓ cotton rolls
- ✓ high-volume evacuator
- ✓ saliva ejector

- ✓ air-water tip
- ✓ articulating paper on forceps
- ✓ cotton tip with topical
- ✓ anesthetic syringe
- ✓ two Carpules of anesthetic
- ✓ floss
- ✓ endodontic ruler

After tray set-up is complete, the dental assistant will set up the following:

- ✻ Handpieces: high-speed with fissure bur (e.g., #56) prerun with water and fiberoptics on
  slow-speed with Gates-Glidden burs and rotary instruments ready
- ✻ Anesthetic: 30-gauge needle for maxillary and children
  27- or 30-gauge needle for mandibular, depending on doctor's preference
- ✻ Periapical radiographs in viewbox
- ✻ Precut dental dam with one hole only and appropriate clamp
- ✻ Slip of paper with working lengths and corresponding files

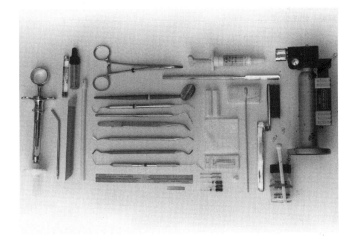

Figure 1-10. Standard tray setup for root canal obturation procedure. Note the Gates-Glidden burs, broaches, and files, heat source, gutta percha cones, and root canal sealer.

✳ Sodium hypochlorite, hydrogen peroxide, and irrigating syringe
✳ Files and reamers (#08–#70) in sponge
✳ Broaches, paper points (medium and fine), cotton pellets, CAVIT, x-ray film, gutta percha cones, heat source, Schilder pluggers (#8–#10), root canal sealer, spatula, matches

Seating Patient

The dental assistant:

✳ Greets the patient, places the bib, and discusses the appointment with the patient
✳ Asks the patient if there are any changes in his or her health history
✳ Makes chart entries and has notepad ready to write notes
✳ Places topical in correct area and summons the doctor

Examination

The dental assistant:

✳ Has mouth mirror, explorer, and treatment plan ready
✳ Passes anesthetic syringe to the doctor

Isolation

The dental assistant:

✳ Places the dental dam (only need one hole)

Preparation and Fill

The doctor:

- ✳ Removes the temporary in the access cavity
- ✳ Tries in all files at final working length
- ✳ Irrigates and dries canal(s) with paper points
- ✳ Tries in gutta percha cone to working length and then trims apex of cone by 0.5 mm
- ✳ Seats the gutta percha cone with root canal sealer
- ✳ Sears off gutta percha cone with hot plugger and condenses with Schilder pluggers
- ✳ Backfills with additional gutta percha cones or warm gutta percha source (e.g., OBTURA)

The dental assistant:

- ✳ Takes final radiograph
- ✳ Places temporary filling in access or prepares for post buildup procedure

Finish

The dental assistant:

- ✳ Provides postoperative instructions as directed by the doctor
- ✳ Rinses the patient after removal of the dental dam
- ✳ Checks occlusion with 2×2s and articulating paper on forceps
- ✳ Finishes chart entry and asks the doctor for the next appointment
- ✳ Removes the bib and walks the patient to the front desk

The dental assistant will now remove all the plastic barriers in the operatory, replace them with new ones, and spray all contaminated surfaces with an OSHA-approved disinfectant to get the operatory ready for the next patient.

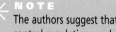
NOTE
The authors suggest that users of this text review their current state infection control regulations and modify these procedures if necessary.

Post Buildup Procedure

Operatory Preparation

Barriers

Prior to seating the patient, the dental assistant will place appropriate infection control barriers in the operatory. These include plastic covering for all surfaces that may become contaminated and that will not be disinfected with an aerosol spray following the procedure. Such surfaces may include

- overhead light handles and light switches
- operatory delivery systems
- plastic tubing for handpieces and suction
- nitrous oxide equipment
- x-ray heads
- doctor and assistant stools
- headrest on the dental chair

Personal protective equipment (eyewear, masks, and gloves) will be available and ready to use during the procedure for both the doctor and the dental assistant. Protective eyewear will also be provided for the patient.

Amalgam or Composite Tray (Fig. 1-11A)

- ✓ instruments (mouth mirror, explorer, periodontal probe, cotton pliers, spoon excavator, hemostats)
- ✓ 2×2s
- ✓ cotton rolls
- ✓ high-volume evacuator
- ✓ saliva ejector
- ✓ air-water tip
- ✓ articulating paper on forceps
- ✓ cotton tip with topical
- ✓ anesthetic syringe
- ✓ two Carpules of anesthetic
- ✓ matrix bands
- ✓ wedges, floss

After tray setup is complete, the dental assistant will set up the following:

* Handpieces: high-speed with fissure bur (e.g., #56) prerun with water and fiberoptics on
  slow-speed with round bur (e.g., #6) and Gates-Glidden burs ready
* Anesthetic: 30-gauge needle for maxillary and children
  27- or 30-gauge needle for mandibular, depending on doctor's preference
* If composite: have all the above ready plus auto-cure composite material, mixing pad, post kit, composite finishing material (Fig. 1-11B).
* Tofflemire matrix bands
* Precut dental dam and appropriate clamp
* Periapical radiographs in viewbox

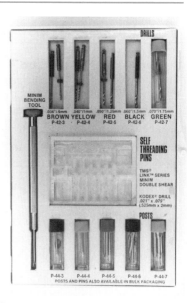

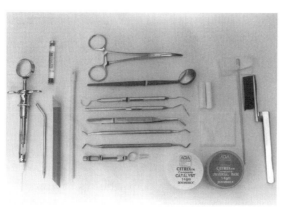

A   **B**

Figure 1-11. (**A**) Standard tray setup for post buildup procedure. Included are a Tofflemire matrix and retainer, wedges, and core buildup material. (**B**) Post kit containing drills, pins, posts, and bending tool.

Seating Patient

The dental assistant:

- ✳ Greets the patient, places the bib, and discusses the appointment with the patient
- ✳ Asks the patient if there are any changes in his or her health history
- ✳ Makes chart entries and has notepad ready to write notes
- ✳ Places topical in correct area and summons the doctor

Examination

The dental assistant:

- ✳ Has mouth mirror, explorer, and treatment plan ready
- ✳ Passes anesthetic syringe to the doctor

Isolation

The dental assistant:

- ✳ Places the dental dam with the appropriate clamp
- ✳ Has the composite and post kit ready

Preparation

The doctor:

✳ Prepares the tooth and removes the temporary with high-speed handpiece and fissure bur, removes the decay with slow-speed handpiece and round bur, and prepares the post space with a post kit (e.g., PARAPOST)
✳ Cuts post with post cutters and tries in with hemostats or cotton pliers
✳ Seats post with cement (e.g., zinc phosphate or glass ionomer)

The dental assistant places the matrix band and wedges.

Fill

The doctor:

✳ Fills tooth with designated buildup material (amalgam or composite)
✳ Trims and/or carves the restoration

Finish

The dental assistant:

✳ Provides postoperative instructions as directed by the doctor
✳ Rinses the patient after removal of the dental dam
✳ Finishes the chart entry while the doctor checks the occlusion with 2×2s and articulating paper on forceps and asks the doctor for the next appointment
✳ Removes the bib and walks the patient to the front desk

The dental assistant will now remove all the plastic barriers in the operatory, replace them with new ones, and spray all contaminated surfaces with an OSHA-approved disinfectant to get the operatory ready for the next patient.

 NOTE
The authors suggest that users of this text review their current state infection control regulations and modify these procedures if necessary.

Cast Post and Core Procedure

Operatory Preparation

Barriers

Prior to seating the patient, the dental assistant will place appropriate infection control barriers in the operatory. These include plastic covering for all surfaces that may become contaminated and that will not be disinfected with an aerosol spray following the procedure. Such surfaces may include

- overhead light handles and light switches
- operatory delivery systems
- plastic tubing for handpieces and suction
- nitrous oxide equipment
- x-ray heads
- doctor and assistant stools
- headrest on the dental chair

Personal protective equipment (eyewear, masks, and gloves) will be available and ready to use during the procedure for both the doctor and the dental assistant. Protective eyewear will also be provided for the patient.

Crown and Bridge Tray (Fig. 1-12)

- ✓ instruments (mouth mirror, explorer, periodontal probe, cotton pliers, spoon excavator, retraction cord placing instruments, plastic instrument, hemostats)
- ✓ 2×2s
- ✓ cotton rolls
- ✓ high-volume evacuator
- ✓ saliva ejector
- ✓ air-water tip
- ✓ articulating paper on forceps
- ✓ cotton tip with topical
- ✓ anesthetic syringe
- ✓ two Carpules of anesthetic
- ✓ dental dam setup and clamps
- ✓ post kit
- ✓ floss

After tray setup is complete, the dental assistant will set up the following:

* Handpieces: high-speed with crown prep diamond prerun with water and fiberoptics on
  slow-speed with straight nose cone and acrylic bur
* Anesthetic: 30-gauge needle for maxillary and children
  27- or 30-gauge needle for mandibular, depending on doctor's preference
* Precut dental dam and appropriate clamp
* Final fill endodontic periapical radiograph in viewbox
* Dappen dish with hemostatic agent

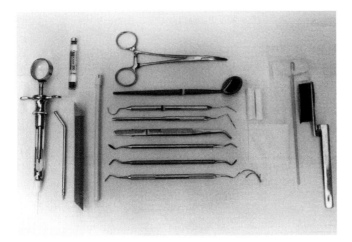

Figure 1-12. Standard tray setup for a cast post and core procedure. Note the retraction cord and placing instrument.

✳ Precut retraction cord of appropriate size
✳ Final impression material and impression syringe
✳ Custom or perforated acrylic trays and tray adhesive
✳ Premeasured alginate and water, spatula and bowl, and stock metal tray for opposing impression
✳ Bite registration material
✳ Dappen dish with acrylic
✳ Vacuform shell, ION, polycarbonate, etc., for temporary crown
✳ Temporary cement on pad with spatula
✳ Lab prescription forms and shade guide

Seating Patient

The dental assistant:

✳ Greets the patient, places the bib, and discusses the appointment with the patient
✳ Asks the patient if there are any changes in his or her health history
✳ Takes wax bite for temporary if tooth is not broken
✳ Tries in impression trays for final impression and opposing model to check fit
✳ Makes chart entries and has notepad ready to write notes
✳ Places topical in correct area and summons the doctor

Examination

The dental assistant:

* Has mouth mirror, explorer, and treatment plan ready
* Passes anesthetic syringe to the doctor

Isolation

The dental assistant:

* Places the dental dam with the appropriate clamp

Preparation

The doctor:

* Removes the temporary and prepares the tooth with the high-speed hand-piece, and removes decay with the slow-speed handpiece and round bur
* Prepares the post space with slow-speed handpiece and drill from post kit
* Cuts the plastic post with scissors and tries in with hemostats or cotton pliers

The dental assistant:

* Places the retraction cord under the doctor's supervision
* Removes the dental dam and rinses the patient
* Takes the opposing arch impression with alginate in stock metal tray

The doctor:

* Takes the final impression with the plastic post in the canal
* Takes bite registration

The dental assistant fabricates the temporary crown, using the aluminum post in the canal from the post kit (see the section "Temporary Crown Fabrication Procedure" for explanation).

Finish

The dental assistant:

* Checks the occlusion on the temporary crown with 2×2s and articulating paper on forceps
* Cements the temporary crown with temporary cement
* Removes excess cement and flosses around the temporary crown

✳ Rinses the patient and provides postoperative instructions as directed by
   the doctor
✳ Finishes the chart entries and lab prescription forms
✳ Removes the bib and walks the patient to the front desk

The dental assistant will now remove all the plastic barriers in the operatory, replace them with new ones, and spray all contaminated surfaces with an OSHA-
approved disinfectant to get the operatory ready for the next patient.

NOTE
The authors suggest that users of this text review their current state infection
control regulations and modify these procedures if necessary.

Removable Partial Dentures (Preparation and Impression)

In the following sections on removable partial and complete dentures, the authors assume that initial impressions, facebow transfer, and centric relation records have been taken previously at the adult initial examination. From these, the authors have accurately mounted study casts to evaluate occlusion, design partial denture frameworks, and prepare custom acrylic final impression trays for complete dentures.

Operatory Preparation

Barriers

Prior to seating the patient, the dental assistant will place appropriate infection control barriers in the operatory. These include plastic covering for all surfaces that may become contaminated and that will not be disinfected with an aerosol spray following the procedure. Such surfaces may include

- overhead light handles and light switches
- operatory delivery systems
- plastic tubing for handpieces and suction
- nitrous oxide equipment
- x-ray heads
- doctor and assistant stools
- headrest on the dental chair

Personal protective equipment (eyewear, masks, and gloves) will be available and ready to use during the procedure for both the doctor and the dental assistant. Protective eyewear will also be provided for the patient.

Exam Tray

- ✓ instruments (mouth mirror, explorer, periodontal probe, cotton pliers)
- ✓ 2×2s
- ✓ cotton rolls
- ✓ high-volume evacuator
- ✓ saliva ejector
- ✓ air-water tip
- ✓ articulating paper on forceps

After tray setup is complete, the dental assistant will set up the following:

- ✱ Handpieces: high-speed with straight diamond prerun with water and fiberoptics on, and white stone and #6 round bur ready
- ✱ Panoramic, full mouth series, bitewing, and/or periapical radiographs in viewbox

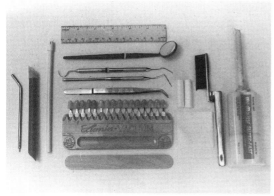 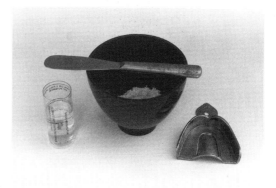

A   **B**

Figure 1-13. (**A**) Standard tray setup for removable partial denture initial impression procedure. Included is the VITA shade guide, ruler, and bite registration material. (**B**) Premeasured water and alginate, spatula, mixing bowl, and stock metal impression tray.

* Premeasured alginate and water, spatula and bowl, impression trays, bite registration materials, ruler, tongue blades, lab prescription forms, shade guide (Fig. 1-13A,B).

Seating Patient

The dental assistant:

* Greets the patient, places the bib, and discusses the appointment with the patient
* Asks the patient if there are any changes in his or her health history
* Chooses shade and records in chart, to be confirmed later with the doctor
* Tries in impression trays for final impression and opposing model to check fit
* Makes chart entries, has notepad ready to write notes, and summons the doctor

Examination and Isolation

The dental assistant:

* Has mouth mirror, explorer, and treatment plan ready
* Has cotton rolls ready

Preparation

The doctor:

* Prepares guide planes and rest seats, then polishes these surfaces

* Checks the occlusion with 2×2s and articulating paper on forceps
* Takes final impression with selected final impression material and tray
* Takes bite registration with bite registration material
* Selects the teeth (shade and mould) and verifies with the patient

The dental assistant:

* Takes opposing arch impression with alginate in stock metal tray

Finish

The dental assistant:

* Rinses the patient and asks the doctor for the next appointment
* Finishes the chart entries and lab prescription forms
* Removes the bib and walks the patient to the front desk

The dental assistant will now remove all the plastic barriers in the operatory, replace them with new ones, and spray all contaminated surfaces with an OSHA-approved disinfectant to get the operatory ready for the next patient.

> **NOTE**
> The authors suggest that users of this text review their current state infection control regulations and modify these procedures if necessary.

Removable Partial Dentures (Framework Try-In)

Operatory Preparation

Barriers

Prior to seating the patient, the dental assistant will place appropriate infection control barriers in the operatory. These include plastic covering for all surfaces that may become contaminated and that will not be disinfected with an aerosol spray following the procedure. Such surfaces may include

- overhead light handles and light switches
- operatory delivery systems
- plastic tubing for handpieces and suction
- nitrous oxide equipment
- x-ray heads
- doctor and assistant stools
- headrest on the dental chair

Personal protective equipment (eyewear, masks, and gloves) will be available and ready to use during the procedure for both the doctor and the dental assistant. Protective eyewear will also be provided for the patient.

Exam Tray (Fig. 1-14)

- ✓ instruments (mouth mirror, explorer, periodontal probe, cotton pliers)
- ✓ 2×2s
- ✓ cotton rolls
- ✓ high-volume evacuator
- ✓ saliva ejector
- ✓ air-water tip
- ✓ articulating paper on forceps

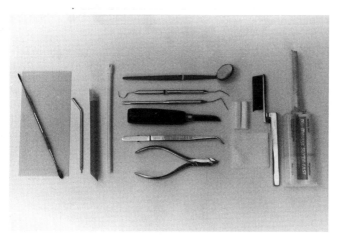

Figure 1-14. Standard tray setup for removable partial denture framework try-in procedure. Note the pink baseplate wax, wax spatula, and orthodontic three-prong pliers.

After tray setup is complete, the dental assistant will set up the following:

✳ Handpieces: high-speed with straight diamond prerun with water and fiberoptics on
slow-speed with straight nose cone and Joe Dandy disc and burlew wheel ready

✳ Panoramic, full mouth series, bitewing, and/or periapical radiographs in viewbox

✳ Pink baseplate wax and wax spatula, materials for bite registration (e.g. ALUWAX and REGISIL 2X), large putty knife, lab knife, matches, lab prescription forms, Hanau torch and water bath, orthodontic pliers (three-prong)

Seating Patient

The dental assistant:

✳ Greets the patient, places the bib, and discusses the appointment with the patient

✳ Asks the patient if there are any changes in his or her health history

✳ Makes chart entries, has notepad ready to write notes, and summons the doctor

Examination and Isolation

The dental assistant:

✳ Has mouth mirror, explorer, and treatment plan ready

✳ Has cotton rolls ready

Preparation

The doctor:

✳ Seats the partial denture framework

✳ Records maxillary/mandibular relations with bite registration material and/or baseplate wax

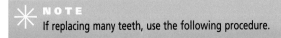

✳ **NOTE**
If replacing many teeth, use the following procedure.

The doctor:

* ✳ Establishes vertical dimension of rest
* ✳ Establishes vertical dimension of occlusion
* ✳ Establishes closest speaking space
* ✳ Establishes tooth-to-lip relationship
* ✳ Evaluates overjet
* ✳ Marks and records midline

Finish

The doctor has the patient sign the chart stating satisfaction with the set-up and esthetics before processing.

The dental assistant:

* ✳ Rinses the patient and asks the doctor for the next appointment

NOTE
If replacing many teeth, have clinical try-in.

* ✳ Finishes the chart entries and lab prescription forms
* ✳ Removes the bib and walks the patient to the front desk

The dental assistant will now remove all the plastic barriers in the operatory, replace them with new ones, and spray all contaminated surfaces with an OSHA-approved disinfectant to get the operatory ready for the next patient.

NOTE
The authors suggest that users of this text review their current state infection control regulations and modify these procedures if necessary.

Removable Partial Dentures (Delivery and Postop)

Operatory Preparation

Barriers

Prior to seating the patient, the dental assistant will place appropriate infection control barriers in the operatory. These include plastic covering for all surfaces that may become contaminated and that will not be disinfected with an aerosol spray following the procedure. Such surfaces may include

- overhead light handles and light switches
- operatory delivery systems
- plastic tubing for handpieces and suction
- nitrous oxide equipment
- x-ray heads
- doctor and assistant stools
- headrest on the dental chair

Personal protective equipment (eyewear, masks, and gloves) will be available and ready to use during the procedure for both the doctor and the dental assistant. Protective eyewear will also be provided for the patient.

Exam Tray (Fig. 1-15)

- ✓ instruments (mouth mirror, explorer, periodontal probe, cotton pliers)
- ✓ 2×2s
- ✓ cotton rolls
- ✓ high-volume evacuator
- ✓ saliva ejector
- ✓ air-water tip
- ✓ articulating paper on forceps

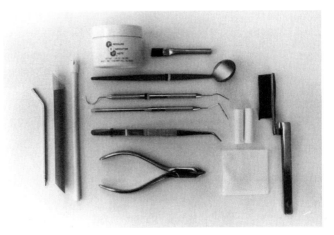

Figure 1-15. Standard tray setup for removable partial denture delivery procedure. Note the orthodontic three-prong pliers, pressure indicator paste, and brush.

After tray setup is complete, the dental assistant will set up the following:

 ✳ Handpieces: high-speed with straight diamond prerun with water and fiberoptics on
   slow-speed with straight nose cone and acrylic bur
 ✳ Panoramic, full mouth series, bitewing and/or periapical radiographs in viewbox
 ✳ Pressure indicator paste and brushes, orthodontic pliers (three-prong)

Seating Patient

The dental assistant:

 ✳ Greets the patient, places the bib, and discusses the appointment with the patient
 ✳ Asks the patient if there are any changes in his or her health history
 ✳ Makes chart entries, has notepad ready to write notes, and summons the doctor

Examination and Isolation

The dental assistant:

 ✳ Has mouth mirror, explorer, and treatment plan ready
 ✳ Has cotton rolls ready

Preparation and Finish

The doctor:

 ✳ Seats the partial denture and adjusts discrepancies in the framework
 ✳ Checks the occlusion with 2×2s and articulating paper on forceps

The dental assistant:

 ✳ Explains postoperative instructions and how to care for the denture, as instructed by the doctor
 ✳ Finishes the chart entry and asks the doctor for the next appointment
 ✳ Removes the bib and walks the patient to the front desk

The dental assistant will now remove all the plastic barriers in the operatory, replace them with new ones, and spray all contaminated surfaces with an OSHA-approved disinfectant to get the operatory ready for the next patient.

 N O T E
The authors suggest that users of this text review their current state infection control regulations and modify these procedures if necessary.

Complete Dentures (Final Impressions)

In the following sections on complete dentures, the authors assume that initial impressions, facebow transfer, and centric relation records have been taken previously at the adult initial examination. From these, the authors have accurately mounted study casts to evaluate occlusion and have prepared custom acrylic final impression trays for complete dentures.

Operatory Preparation

Barriers

Prior to seating the patient, the dental assistant will place appropriate infection control barriers in the operatory. These include plastic covering for all surfaces that may become contaminated and that will not be disinfected with an aerosol spray following the procedure. Such surfaces may include

- overhead light handles and light switches
- operatory delivery systems
- plastic tubing for handpieces and suction
- nitrous oxide equipment
- x-ray heads
- doctor and assistant stools
- headrest on the dental chair

Personal protective equipment (eyewear, masks, and gloves) will be available and ready to use during the procedure for both the doctor and the dental assistant. Protective eyewear will also be provided for the patient.

Exam Tray (Fig. 1-16)

- ✓ instruments (mouth mirror, periodontal probe, cotton pliers)
- ✓ 2×2s
- ✓ cotton rolls
- ✓ high-volume evacuator
- ✓ saliva ejector
- ✓ air-water tip

After tray setup is complete, the dental assistant will set up the following:

* Handpieces: slow-speed with straight nose cone and acrylic bur
* Panoramic radiograph in viewbox
* Spatulas, final impression material, custom impression trays, bite registra-

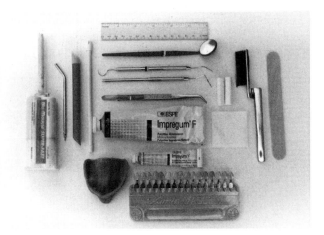

Figure 1-16. Standard tray setup for complete denture final impression procedure. Included are final impression material, custom acrylic impression tray, bite registration material, ruler, tongue blade, and shade guide.

tion material, ruler, tongue blades, lab prescription forms, shade guide (e.g., VITA), mould guide

Seating Patient

The dental assistant:

* Greets the patient, places the bib, and discusses the appointment with the patient
* Asks the patient if there are any changes in his or her health history
* Makes chart entries, has notepad ready, and summons the doctor

Exam, Isolation, and Preparation

The dental assistant:

* Has the mouth mirror and treatment plan ready
* Tries in final impression trays

The doctor:

* Takes final impression with final impression material in custom acrylic trays
* Selects teeth (shade and mould)

Finish

The dental assistant:

* Finishes the chart entry and asks the doctor for the next appointment
* Removes the bib and walks the patient to the front desk

The dental assistant will now remove all the plastic barriers in the operatory, replace them with new ones, and spray all contaminated surfaces with an OSHA-approved disinfectant to get the operatory ready for the next patient.

 N O T E
The authors suggest that users of this text review their current state infection control regulations and modify these procedures if necessary.

Complete Dentures (Maxillary–Mandibular Relations)

Operatory Preparation

Barriers

Prior to seating the patient, the dental assistant will place appropriate infection control barriers in the operatory. These include plastic covering for all surfaces that may become contaminated and that will not be disinfected with an aerosol spray following the procedure. Such surfaces may include

- overhead light handles and light switches
- operatory delivery systems
- plastic tubing for handpieces and suction
- nitrous oxide equipment
- x-ray heads
- doctor and assistant stools
- headrest on the dental chair

Personal protective equipment (eyewear, masks, and gloves) will be available and ready to use during the procedure for both the doctor and the dental assistant. Protective eyewear will also be provided for the patient.

Exam Tray (Fig. 1-17)

✓ instruments (mouth mirror, periodontal probe, cotton pliers)
✓ 2×2s
✓ cotton rolls, high-volume evacuator
✓ saliva ejector
✓ air-water tip

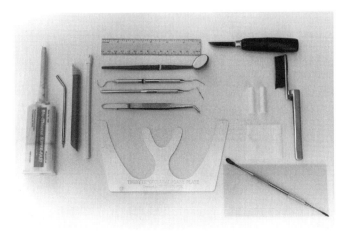

Figure 1-17. Standard tray setup for complete denture maxillary–mandibular relations records procedure. Included are bite registration material, pink baseplate wax, wax spatula, lab knife, ruler, and occlusal plane guide.

After tray setup is complete, the dental assistant will set up the following:

✳ Handpieces: slow-speed with straight nose cone and acrylic bur
✳ Panoramic radiograph in viewbox
✳ Pink baseplate wax and wax spatula, bite registration material, large putty knife, lab knife, matches, lab prescription forms, Hanau torch and water bath, ruler, occlusal plane guide

Seating Patient

The dental assistant:

✳ Greets the patient, places the bib, and discusses the appointment with the patient
✳ Asks the patient if there are any changes in his or her health history
✳ Makes chart entries, has notepad ready, and summons the doctor

Exam, Isolation, and Preparation

The dental assistant:

✳ Has the mouth mirror and treatment plan ready

The doctor:

✳ Tries in maxillary and mandibular occlusion rims and evaluates fit
✳ Establishes Camper's plane and smile line
✳ Establishes vertical dimension of rest (say "Mom")
✳ Establishes vertical dimension of occlusion (−3 mm)
✳ Establishes closest speaking space (say "cheese")
✳ Evaluates tooth–lip relation (say "fifty-five")
✳ Evaluates overjet
✳ Marks midline on wax rims
✳ Establishes maxillary–mandibular relations with bite registration material in centric relation

Finish

The dental assistant:

✳ Finishes the chart entry and lab forms and asks the doctor for the next appointment
✳ Removes the bib and walks the patient to the front desk

The dental assistant will now remove all the plastic barriers in the operatory, replace them with new ones, and spray all contaminated surfaces with an OSHA-approved disinfectant to get the operatory ready for the next patient.

NOTE
The authors suggest that users of this text review their current state infection control regulations and modify these procedures if necessary.

Complete Dentures (Clinical Wax Try-In)

Operatory Preparation

Barriers

Prior to seating the patient, the dental assistant will place appropriate infection control barriers in the operatory. These include plastic covering for all surfaces that may become contaminated and that will not be disinfected with an aerosol spray following the procedure. Such surfaces may include

- overhead light handles and light switches
- operatory delivery systems
- plastic tubing for handpieces and suction
- nitrous oxide equipment
- x-ray heads
- doctor and assistant stools
- headrest on the dental chair

Personal protective equipment (eyewear, masks, and gloves) will be available and ready to use during the procedure for both the doctor and the dental assistant. Protective eyewear will also be provided for the patient.

Exam Tray

✓ instruments (mouth mirror, periodontal probe, cotton pliers)
✓ 2×2s
✓ cotton rolls
✓ high-volume evacuator
✓ saliva ejector
✓ air-water tip

After tray setup is complete, the dental assistant will set up the following:

* Handpieces: slow-speed with straight nose cone and acrylic bur
* Panoramic radiograph in viewbox
* Pink baseplate wax and wax spatula, bite registration material, large putty knife, lab knife, matches, lab prescription forms, Hanau torch and water bath, ruler, occlusal plane guide

Seating Patient

The dental assistant:

* Greets the patient, places the bib, and discusses the appointment with the patient

* Asks the patient if there are any changes in his or her health history
* Makes chart entries, has notepad ready, and summons the doctor

Exam, Isolation, and Preparation

The dental assistant:

* Has the mouth mirror and treatment plan ready

The doctor:

* Tries in maxillary and/or mandibular denture (in wax) and evaluates fit
* Establishes vertical dimension of rest (say "Mom")
* Establishes vertical dimension of occlusion (-3 mm)
* Establishes closest speaking space (say "cheese")
* Evaluates tooth–lip relation (say "fifty-five")
* Evaluates overjet
* Marks midline on wax rims
* Evaluates maxillary–mandibular relations with wax setups and takes bite registration in centric relation if necessary
* Evaluates smile line

Finish

The doctor has the patient sign in the chart that the setup is satisfactory prior to processing of the dentures.

The dental assistant:

* Finishes the chart entry and lab forms and asks the doctor for the next appointment
* Removes the bib and walks the patient to the front desk

The dental assistant will now remove all the plastic barriers in the operatory, replace them with new ones, and spray all contaminated surfaces with an OSHA-approved disinfectant to get the operatory ready for the next patient.

NOTE
The authors suggest that users of this text review their current state infection control regulations and modify these procedures if necessary.

Complete Dentures (Delivery and Postop)

Operatory Preparation

Barriers

Prior to seating the patient, the dental assistant will place appropriate infection control barriers in the operatory. These include plastic covering for all surfaces that may become contaminated and that will not be disinfected with an aerosol spray following the procedure. Such surfaces may include

- overhead light handles and light switches
- operatory delivery systems
- plastic tubing for handpieces and suction

- nitrous oxide equipment
- x-ray heads
- doctor and assistant stools
- headrest on the dental chair

Personal protective equipment (eyewear, masks, and gloves) will be available and ready to use during the procedure for both the doctor and the dental assistant. Protective eyewear will also be provided for the patient.

Exam Tray (Fig. 1-18)

- ✓ instruments (mouth mirror, periodontal probe, cotton pliers)
- ✓ 2×2s
- ✓ cotton rolls

- ✓ high-volume evacuator
- ✓ saliva ejector
- ✓ air-water tip
- ✓ articulating paper on forceps

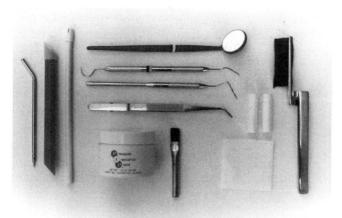

Figure 1-18. Standard tray setup for complete denture delivery procedure. Included are articulating paper on forceps, pressure indicator paste, and brush.

After tray setup is complete, the dental assistant will set up the following:

- ✳ Handpieces: slow-speed with straight nose cone and acrylic bur
- ✳ Panoramic radiograph in viewbox
- ✳ Pressure indicator paste and brush, Thompson pencil

Seating Patient

The dental assistant:

- ✳ Greets the patient, places the bib, and discusses the appointment with the patient
- ✳ Asks the patient if there are any changes in his or her health history
- ✳ Makes chart entries, has notepad ready, and summons the doctor

Exam, Isolation, and Preparation

The dental assistant:

- ✳ Has the mouth mirror and treatment plan ready

The doctor:

- ✳ Tries in maxillary and/or mandibular denture, evaluates fit, and adjusts any sore spots using pressure indicator paste
- ✳ Adjusts the occlusion with articulating paper on forceps and 2×2s

The dental assistant polishes the denture.

Finish

The dental assistant:

- ✳ Explains postoperative instructions and how to care for the denture, as instructed by the doctor
- ✳ Finishes the chart entry and lab forms and asks the doctor for the next appointment
- ✳ Removes the bib and walks the patient to the front desk

The dental assistant will now remove all the plastic barriers in the operatory, replace them with new ones, and spray all contaminated surfaces with an OSHA-approved disinfectant to get the operatory ready for the next patient.

 NOTE
The authors suggest that users of this text review their current state infection control regulations and modify these procedures if necessary.

ERA Attachment Fabrication Procedure

(The patient already has a lower complete denture fabricated, with two teeth previously receiving root canal treatment, e.g., #22 and #27.)

Operatory Preparation

Barriers

Prior to seating the patient, the dental assistant will place the appropriate infection control barriers in the operatory. These include plastic covering for all surfaces that may become contaminated and that will not be disinfected with an aerosol spray following the procedure. Such surfaces may include

- overhead light handles and light switches
- operatory delivery systems
- plastic tubing for handpieces and suction

- nitrous oxide equipment
- x-ray heads
- doctor and assistant stools
- headrest on the dental chair

Personal protective equipment (eyewear, masks, and gloves) will be available and ready to use during the procedure for both the doctor and the dental assistant. Protective eyewear will also be provided for the patient.

Exam Tray (Fig. 1-19)

- ✓ instruments (mouth mirror, explorer, periodontal probe, cotton pliers)
- ✓ 2×2s
- ✓ cotton rolls
- ✓ high-volume evacuator
- ✓ saliva ejector
- ✓ air-water tip
- ✓ cotton tip with topical

- ✓ anesthetic syringe
- ✓ two Carpules anesthetic
- ✓ dappen dish
- ✓ spatula
- ✓ ERA attachment kit and materials
- ✓ post kit
- ✓ separating media
- ✓ cold cure acrylic
- ✓ benda brushes

After tray setup is complete, the dental assistant will set up the following:

* Handpieces: high-speed with diamond bur prerun with water and fiberoptics on

slow-speed with post drill and straight nose cone with acrylic bur ready

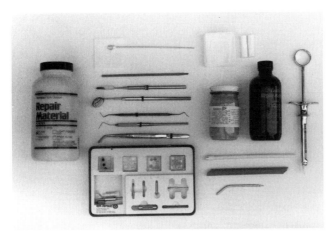

Figure 1-19. Standard tray setup for ERA attachment procedure. Included are a mixing spatula, cold cure acrylic, separating medium, benda brush, and ERA kit.

✳ Anesthetic: 30-gauge needle for maxillary

27- or 30-gauge needle for mandibular, depending on doctor's preference

✳ Periapical radiographs of completed root canals in viewbox
✳ Dappen dishes with pink cold cure acrylic and monomer

Seating Patient

The dental assistant:

✳ Greets the patient, places the bib, and discusses the appointment with the patient
✳ Asks the patient if there are any changes in his or her health history
✳ Asks the patient if there are any sore spots with the dentures and has pressure indicator paste ready for the doctor
✳ Makes chart entries and has notepad ready to write notes
✳ Places topical in correct area (if indicated) and summons the doctor

Examination

The dental assistant:

✳ Has mouth mirror, explorer, and treatment plan ready
✳ Passes anesthetic syringe to the doctor (if indicated by the doctor)

Isolation

The dental assistant:

✳ Places the Svedopter or cotton rolls at doctor's request

Preparation

The doctor:

✳ Prepares the abutment teeth down to tissue level (e.g., #22 and #27)
✳ Drills pilot holes with post drill
✳ Countersinks with slow-speed handpiece and water
✳ Fits and cuts male ERA post
✳ Cements ERA post with cement while keeping male attachments parallel
✳ Removes excess cement and rounds off abutment teeth with diamond finishing bur
✳ Places black nylon seating caps on male ERA posts
✳ Places holes into under side of denture (lingual to the teeth) so that the denture seats without touching sides of abutment teeth and black seating caps

The dental assistant:

✳ Paints separating media within 2 mm of hole on under side and top side of lower denture
✳ Places monomer around holes and black seating caps
✳ Mixes acrylic and fills holes

The doctor:

✳ Seats the denture and lets the excess acrylic ooze out, removes the excess, and lets the patient close in a normal bite and sit for 9 minutes while the assistant rinses the patient's mouth with cold water
✳ Removes the lower denture from the male ERA abutment teeth with a mouth mirror handle and trims the excess undercuts
✳ Drills out the black seating caps and puts new orange ones in
✳ Checks occlusion with 2×2s and articulating paper on forceps
✳ Has the dental assistant polish the lower denture

Finish

The dental assistant:

✳ Reviews the postoperative instructions and procedure with the patient
✳ Rinses the patient

✳ Finishes the chart entry and asks the doctor for the next appointment

✳ Removes the bib and walks the patient to the front desk

The dental assistant will now remove all the plastic barriers in the operatory, replace them with new ones, and spray all contaminated surfaces with an OSHA-approved disinfectant to get the operatory ready for the next patient.

NOTE
The authors suggest that users of this text review their current state infection control regulations and modify these procedures if necessary.

Periodontal Scaling and Polish

Operatory Preparation

Barriers

Prior to seating the patient, the dental assistant will place the appropriate infection control barriers in the operatory. These include plastic covering for all surfaces that may become contaminated and that will not be disinfected with an aerosol spray following the procedure. Such surfaces may include

- overhead light handles and light switches
- operatory delivery systems
- plastic tubing for handpieces and suction
- nitrous oxide equipment
- x-ray heads
- doctor and assistant stools
- headrest on the dental chair

Personal protective equipment (eyewear, masks, and gloves) will be available and ready to use during the procedure for both the doctor and the dental assistant. Protective eyewear will also be provided for the patient.

Curettage Tray (Fig. 1-20)

- ✓ instruments (mouth mirror, explorer, periodontal probe, cotton pliers, various hand scalers, e.g., 4R4L, sickle)
- ✓ 2×2s
- ✓ cotton rolls
- ✓ high-volume evacuator
- ✓ saliva ejector
- ✓ air-water tip
- ✓ cotton tip with topical
- ✓ anesthetic syringe
- ✓ two Carpules of anesthetic
- ✓ floss
- ✓ sonic or ultrasonic scalers
- ✓ prophy paste
- ✓ prophy cup

After tray setup is complete, the dental assistant or hygienist will set up the following:

- ✳ Handpieces: slow-speed with straight nose cone and prophy head
  sonic or ultrasonic scaler if necessary
- ✳ Full mouth series or most current bitewing radiographs in viewbox
- ✳ Anesthetic: 30-gauge needle for maxillary
  27- or 30-gauge needle for mandibular, depending on doctor's preference

Seating Patient

The dental assistant or hygienist:

- ✳ Greets the patient, places the bib, and discusses the appointment with the patient

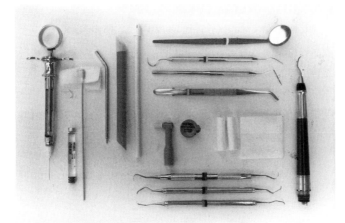

Figure 1-20. Standard tray setup for periodontal scaling, root planing, and maintenance procedures. Included are hand scalers and a sonic scaler handpiece.

✳ Asks the patient if there are any changes in his or her health history
✳ Makes chart entries and has notepad ready to write notes
✳ Places topical in correct area (if indicated) and summons the doctor/hygienist

Examination

The dental assistant:

✳ Has mouth mirror, explorer, and treatment plan ready
✳ Passes anesthetic syringe to the doctor/hygienist (if indicated)

Preparation

The doctor/hygienist:

✳ Scales teeth with mechanical scalers or hand instruments

The dental assistant/hygienist:

✳ Polishes the teeth with prophy paste
✳ Flosses teeth and rinses the patient

Finish

The dental assistant/hygienist:

✳ Discusses oral hygiene instructions and gives patient toothbrush, floss, and periodontal aides

✳ Finishes the chart entry and asks the doctor for the next appointment

✳ Removes the bib and walks the patient to the front desk

The dental assistant will now remove all the plastic barriers in the operatory, replace them with new ones, and spray all contaminated surfaces with an OSHA-approved disinfectant to get the operatory ready for the next patient.

NOTE
The authors suggest that users of this text review their current state infection control regulations and modify these procedures if necessary.

Oral Surgery/Extractions

Operatory Preparation

Barriers

Prior to seating the patient, the dental assistant will place the appropriate infection control barriers in the operatory. These include plastic covering for all surfaces that may become contaminated and that will not be disinfected with an aerosol spray following the procedure. Such surfaces may include

- overhead light handles and light switches
- operatory delivery systems
- plastic tubing for handpieces and suction
- nitrous oxide equipment
- x-ray heads
- doctor and assistant stools
- headrest on the dental chair

Personal protective equipment (eyewear, masks, and gloves) will be available and ready to use during the procedure for both the doctor and the dental assistant. Protective eyewear will also be provided for the patient.

Exam Tray (Fig. 1-21A,B)

- ✓ instruments (mouth mirror, explorer, periodontal probe, cotton pliers)
- ✓ 2×2s
- ✓ cotton rolls
- ✓ high-volume evacuator
- ✓ saliva ejector
- ✓ air-water tip
- ✓ cotton tip with topical
- ✓ anesthetic syringe
- ✓ two Carpules of anesthetic
- ✓ blood pressure equipment
- ✓ retractor(s)
- ✓ surgical curette

After tray setup is complete, the dental assistant will set up the following, as instructed by the doctor:

- ＊ Handpieces: surgical high-speed with a surgical-length fissure bur
- ＊ Full mouth series, panoramic, or periapical radiographs in viewbox
- ＊ Elevators (e.g., 34, 301 and periosteal elevators)
- ＊ Bard-Parker blades #12 and #15, blade holder, surgical hemostats, and scissors
- ＊ Irrigating syringe and rinse solution (e.g., Peridex, peroxide, warm water)
- ＊ Forceps (e.g., maxillary: 150, 1, 210s; mandibular: 151, 74, 23, 222, as instructed by the doctor)
- ＊ Postoperative instructions, prescription pad

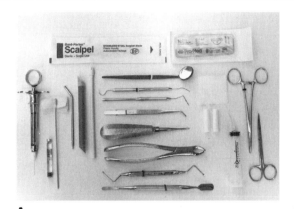
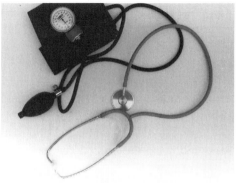

A   **B**

Figure 1-21. (**A**) Standard tray setup for oral surgery procedures. Included are a surgical retractor, surgical curette, elevators, forceps, irrigating syringe, Bard-Parker blades and blade holder, suture material, hemostats, and scissors. (**B**) Blood pressure cuff and stethoscope for oral surgery procedures.

✳ Anesthetic: 30-gauge needle for maxillary and children
27- or 30-gauge needle for mandibular, depending on doctor's preference
✳ Sutures and needle holder

Seating Patient

The dental assistant:

✳ Greets the patient, places the bib, and discusses the appointment with the patient
✳ Takes blood pressure
✳ Takes periapical radiograph if necessary
✳ Asks the patient if there are any changes in his or her health history
✳ Makes chart entries and has notepad ready to write notes
✳ Places topical in correct area and summons the doctor

Examination

The dental assistant:

✳ Has mouth mirror, explorer, and treatment plan ready
✳ Passes anesthetic syringe to the doctor

Preparation

The doctor:

- ✳ Tests anesthetic with periosteal elevator or surgical curette, then severs periodontal ligament
- ✳ Elevates tooth with elevators
- ✳ Removes tooth with forceps and places 2×2 gauze pack into socket to control bleeding

Finish

The dental assistant:

- ✳ Discusses and gives postoperative instructions to the patient
- ✳ Replaces damp 2×2 gauze pack with a new one until bleeding is controlled
- ✳ Gives the patient any prescriptions that the doctor has written
- ✳ Finishes the chart entry and asks the doctor for the next appointment
- ✳ Removes the bib and walks the patient to the front desk

The dental assistant will now remove all the plastic barriers in the operatory, replace them with new ones, and spray all contaminated surfaces with an OSHA-approved disinfectant to get the operatory ready for the next patient.

N O T E
The authors suggest that users of this text review their current state infection control regulations and modify these procedures if necessary.

Incision and Drain Procedure

Operatory Preparation

Barriers

Prior to seating the patient, the dental assistant will place the appropriate infection control barriers in the operatory. These include plastic covering for all surfaces that may become contaminated and that will not be disinfected with an aerosol spray following the procedure. Such surfaces may include

- overhead light handles and light switches
- operatory delivery systems
- plastic tubing for handpieces and suction
- nitrous oxide equipment
- x-ray heads
- doctor and assistant stools
- headrest on the dental chair

Personal protective equipment (eyewear, masks, and gloves) will be available and ready to use during the procedure for both the doctor and the dental assistant. Protective eyewear will also be provided for the patient.

Exam Tray (Fig. 1-22)

- ✓ instruments (mouth mirror, explorer, periodontal probe, cotton pliers)
- ✓ 2×2s
- ✓ cotton rolls
- ✓ high-volume evacuator
- ✓ saliva ejector
- ✓ air-water tip
- ✓ cotton tip with topical
- ✓ anesthetic syringe
- ✓ two Carpules of anesthetic
- ✓ surgical curette
- ✓ blood pressure equipment

After tray setup is complete, the dental assistant will set up the following, as instructed by the doctor:

- ✳ Handpieces: surgical high-speed with a surgical-length fissure bur
- ✳ Full mouth series or most current panoramic radiograph in viewbox
- ✳ Bard-Parker blades #12 and #15, blade holder, surgical hemostats, and scissors
- ✳ Irrigating syringe and rinse solution (e.g., Peridex, peroxide, warm water)
- ✳ Postoperative instructions, prescription pad
- ✳ Anesthetic: 30-gauge needle for maxillary and children
      27- or 30-gauge needle for mandibular, depending on doctor's preference
- ✳ Sutures and needle holder

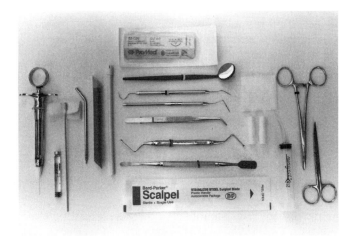

Figure 1-22. Standard tray setup for incision and drainage procedures. Included are a surgical curette, irrigating syringe, Bard-Parker blades and blade holder, suture material, hemostats, and scissors.

Seating Patient

The dental assistant:

✳ Greets the patient, places the bib, and discusses the appointment with the patient
✳ Takes blood pressure
✳ Takes periapical radiograph if necessary
✳ Asks the patient if there are any changes in his or her health history
✳ Makes chart entries and has notepad ready to write notes
✳ Places topical in correct area and summons the doctor

Examination

The dental assistant:

✳ Has mouth mirror, explorer, and treatment plan ready
✳ Passes anesthetic syringe to the doctor

Preparation

The doctor:

✳ Tests anesthetic with periosteal elevator or surgical curette
✳ Opens infected area with a blade while assistant provides suction to the area

* Uses a cotton tip to bring purulence to the surface
* Irrigates the area with an irrigating syringe and rinse solution
* Sutures in drainage "T" for continued drainage if necessary
* Places 2×2 gauze pack to control bleeding if necessary

Finish

The dental assistant:

* Gives postoperative instructions to the patient
* Replaces damp 2×2 gauze pack with a new one until bleeding is controlled
* Gives the patient any prescriptions that the doctor has written
* Finishes the chart entry and asks the doctor for the next appointment
* Removes the bib and walks the patient to the front desk

The dental assistant will now remove all the plastic barriers in the operatory, replace them with new ones, and spray all contaminated surfaces with an OSHA-approved disinfectant to get the operatory ready for the next patient.

 **NOTE**
The authors suggest that users of this text review their current state infection control regulations and modify these procedures if necessary.

Sealant Application Procedure

Operatory Preparation

Barriers

Prior to seating the patient, the dental assistant will place the appropriate infection control barriers in the operatory. These include plastic covering for all surfaces that may become contaminated and that will not be disinfected with an aerosol spray following the procedure. Such surfaces may include

- overhead light handles and light switches
- operatory delivery systems
- plastic tubing for handpieces and suction
- nitrous oxide equipment
- x-ray heads
- doctor and assistant stools
- headrest on the dental chair

Personal protective equipment (eyewear, masks, and gloves) will be available and ready to use during the procedure for both the doctor and the dental assistant. Protective eyewear will also be provided for the patient.

Exam Tray (Fig. 1-23)

- ✓ instruments (mouth mirror, explorer, cotton pliers)
- ✓ 2×2s
- ✓ cotton rolls
- ✓ high-volume evacuator
- ✓ saliva ejector
- ✓ air-water tip
- ✓ articulating paper on forceps
- ✓ absorbent triangles
- ✓ dental dam setup
- ✓ peroxide
- ✓ dappen dish
- ✓ etchant
- ✓ sealant material
- ✓ benda brushes
- ✓ light curing unit

After tray setup is complete, the dental assistant will set up the following:

* Handpieces: high-speed with #330 bur prerun with water and fiber-optics on
slow-speed with prophy brush and cup

Seating Patient

The dental assistant:

* Greets the patient, places the bib, and discusses the appointment with the patient

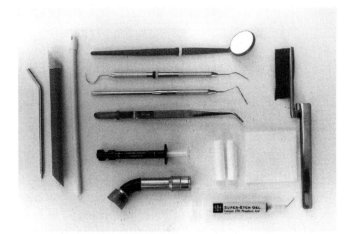

Figure 1-23. Standard tray setup for occlusal sealant application procedure. Pictured at the right are etchant and sealant materials.

✳ Asks the patient if there are any changes in his or her health history
✳ Makes chart entries and has notepad ready to write notes

Examination

The dental assistant:

✳ Has mouth mirror, explorer, and treatment plan ready
✳ Has the doctor check for any pits or grooves to open up with a high-speed handpiece

Isolation

The dental assistant:

✳ Places a dental dam, absorbent triangles, or cotton rolls for isolation

Preparation

The dental assistant:

✳ Cleans debris and saliva from tooth with peroxide, then with brush/cup
✳ Rinses and dries the teeth
✳ Applies etchant from syringe or dappen dish with a benda brush for approximately 10–15 seconds
✳ Rinses tooth for 30 seconds and dries thoroughly

✳ At this point, the enamel should have a chalky appearance and the tooth is ready to be sealed

 N O T E
The authors suggest checking the manufacturer's instructions for etching and curing times.

Fill

The dental assistant:

✳ Applies the sealant material to the dry tooth with a benda brush
✳ With an explorer, moves material around the grooves and removes any bubbles
✳ Light cures directly on the tooth for 20–40 seconds
✳ Tests the sealant for retention with an explorer and removes dental dam, absorbent triangles, or cotton rolls used for isolation
✳ Checks the occlusion with 2×2s and articulating paper on forceps and has the doctor adjust if necessary

Finish

The dental assistant:

✳ Reviews the procedure and any instructions with the patient
✳ Rinses the patient
✳ Finishes the chart entry and asks the doctor for the next appointment
✳ Removes the bib and walks the patient to the front desk

The dental assistant will now remove all the plastic barriers in the operatory, replace them with new ones, and spray all contaminated surfaces with an OSHA-approved disinfectant to get the operatory ready for the next patient.

 N O T E
The authors suggest that users of this text review their current state infection control regulations and modify these procedures if necessary.

Vital Bleaching Tray Fabrication Procedure

Operatory Preparation

Barriers

Prior to seating the patient, the dental assistant will place the appropriate infection control barriers in the operatory. These include plastic covering for all surfaces that may become contaminated and that will not be disinfected with an aerosol spray following the procedure. Such surfaces may include

- overhead light handles and light switches
- operatory delivery systems
- plastic tubing for handpieces and suction
- nitrous oxide equipment
- x-ray heads
- doctor and assistant stools
- headrest on the dental chair

Personal protective equipment (eyewear, masks, and gloves) will be available and ready to use during the procedure for both the doctor and the dental assistant. Protective eyewear will also be provided for the patient.

Exam Tray (Fig. 1-24)

- ✓ instruments (mouth mirror, explorer, periodontal probe, cotton pliers)
- ✓ 2×2s
- ✓ cotton rolls
- ✓ high-volume evacuator
- ✓ saliva ejector
- ✓ air-water tip
- ✓ stock metal impression trays
- ✓ alginate
- ✓ mixing bowls
- ✓ spatulas
- ✓ bleach instruction sheet
- ✓ shade guide

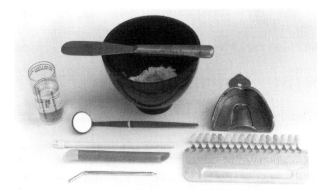

Figure 1-24. Standard tray setup for vital bleaching impression tray fabrication procedure. Included are premeasured alginate and water, spatula and mixing bowl, impression tray, and shade guide.

Seating Patient

The dental assistant:

 ✳ Greets the patient, places the bib, and discusses the appointment with the patient
 ✳ Asks the patient if there are any changes in his or her health history

Examination

The dental assistant:

 ✳ Has mouth mirror, explorer, and treatment plan ready

The doctor:

 ✳ Evaluates the teeth and oral mucosa for susceptibility to the bleaching
 ✳ Takes a prebleaching shade of the teeth

Preparation

The dental assistant:

 ✳ Takes upper and lower alginate impressions
 ✳ Helps the patient with alginate cleanup

Finish

The dental assistant:

 ✳ Reviews the procedure with the patient
 ✳ Rinses the patient
 ✳ Finishes the chart entry and asks the doctor for the next appointment
 ✳ Removes the bib and walks the patient to the front desk
 ✳ Immediately takes the impressions to the lab area, disinfects the impressions, and pours in stone
 ✳ Fabricates trays in lab per individual instructions from manufacturer and doctor (Fig. 1-25)

The dental assistant will now remove all the plastic barriers in the operatory, replace them with new ones, and spray all contaminated surfaces with an OSHA-approved disinfectant to get the operatory ready for the next patient.

NOTE

The authors suggest that users of this text review their current state infection control regulations and modify these procedures if necessary.

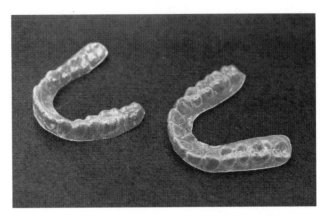

Figure 1-25. Custom-fabricated bleaching trays made with vacuum former ready for insertion.

Vital Bleaching Tray Delivery Procedure

Operatory Preparation

Barriers

Prior to seating the patient, the dental assistant will place the appropriate infection control barriers in the operatory. These include plastic covering for all surfaces that may become contaminated and that will not be disinfected with an aerosol spray following the procedure. Such surfaces may include

- overhead light handles and light switches
- operatory delivery systems
- plastic tubing for handpieces and suction
- nitrous oxide equipment
- x-ray heads
- doctor and assistant stools
- headrest on the dental chair

Personal protective equipment (eyewear, masks, and gloves) will be available and ready to use during the procedure for both the doctor and the dental assistant. Protective eyewear will also be provided for the patient.

Exam Tray (Fig. 1-26)

- ✓ instruments (mouth mirror, explorer, periodontal probe, cotton pliers)
- ✓ 2×2s
- ✓ cotton rolls
- ✓ high-volume evacuator
- ✓ saliva ejector
- ✓ air-water tip
- ✓ shade guide
- ✓ bleaching gel
- ✓ bleaching trays
- ✓ bleaching instruction sheet
- ✓ tray case

Seating Patient

The dental assistant:

* Greets the patient, places the bib, and discusses the appointment with the patient

Preparation

The dental assistant:

* Tries in the bleaching trays, asks the patient if there are any sore areas, and adjusts them as needed
* Records the shade of the patient's teeth in the chart

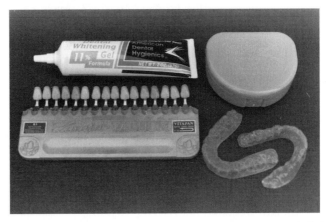

Figure 1-26. Standard tray setup for vital bleaching delivery procedure. Included are the bleaching trays and case and tube of bleaching gel.

✳ Takes a 35mm photo of the patient's teeth (initial photo)
✳ Shows the patient how to administer bleaching gel and how to care for the bleaching trays, and gives the patient a personal tray case

Finish

The dental assistant:

✳ Reviews the procedure and instructions with the patient
✳ Rinses the patient
✳ Finishes the chart entry and asks the doctor for the next appointment
✳ Removes the bib and walks the patient to the front desk

The dental assistant will now remove all the plastic barriers in the operatory, replace them with new ones, and spray all contaminated surfaces with an OSHA-approved disinfectant to get the operatory ready for the next patient.

 NOTE
The authors suggest that users of this text review their current state infection control regulations and modify these procedures if necessary.

Occlusal Splint Records Procedure

Operatory Preparation

Barriers

Prior to seating the patient, the dental assistant will place the appropriate infection control barriers in the operatory. These include plastic covering for all surfaces that may become contaminated and that will not be disinfected with an aerosol spray following the procedure. Such surfaces may include

- overhead light handles and light switches
- operatory delivery systems
- plastic tubing for handpieces and suction
- nitrous oxide equipment
- x-ray heads
- doctor and assistant stools
- headrest on the dental chair

Personal protective equipment (eyewear, masks, and gloves) will be available and ready to use during the procedure for both the doctor and the dental assistant. Protective eyewear will also be provided for the patient.

Exam Tray (Fig. 1-27)

- ✓ instruments (mouth mirror, explorer, periodontal probe, cotton pliers)
- ✓ 2×2s
- ✓ cotton rolls
- ✓ high-volume evacuator
- ✓ saliva ejector
- ✓ air-water tip
- ✓ articulating paper on forceps
- ✓ stock metal impression trays
- ✓ alginate
- ✓ mixing bowl
- ✓ spatula
- ✓ facebow
- ✓ pink wax or a bite registration material
- ✓ anterior central deprogrammer
- ✓ hot water in a mixing bowl

Seating Patient

The dental assistant:

* Greets the patient, places the bib, and discusses the appointment with the patient

Taking Records

The dental assistant:

* Takes upper and lower alginate impressions
* Records facebow transfer and places an anterior deprogrammer in the patient's mouth to relax the muscles (Fig. 1-28A)

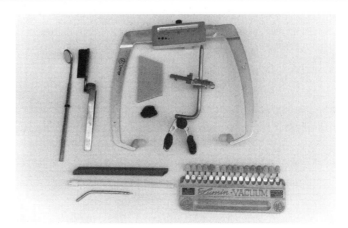

Figure 1-27. Standard tray setup for occlusal splint records procedure. Included are articulating paper on forceps, facebow with bitefork, bite registration material, and anterior central deprogrammer.

The doctor:

✳ Takes bite registration in either wax or a bite registration material after manipulating the patient into centric relation (Fig. 1-28B)

Finish

The dental assistant:

✳ Reviews the procedure and instructions with the patient
✳ Rinses the patient
✳ Finishes the chart entry and asks the doctor for the next appointment
✳ Removes the bib and walks the patient to the front desk
✳ Immediately takes the impressions to the lab area, disinfects the impressions, and pours in stone

The dental assistant will now remove all the plastic barriers in the operatory, replace them with new ones, and spray all contaminated surfaces with an OSHA-approved disinfectant to get the operatory ready for the next patient.

NOTE
The authors suggest that users of this text review their current state infection control regulations and modify these procedures if necessary.

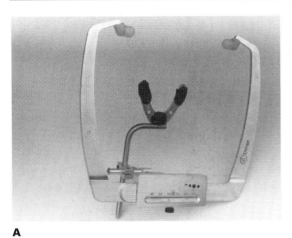
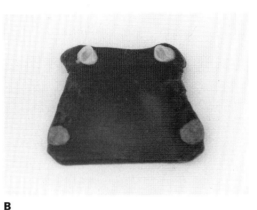

A   **B**

Figure 1-28. (**A**) An example of a facebow transfer with occlusal stops in the anterior and posterior regions. (**B**) An example of a centric relation bite registration made from a Schuyler's wax platform held against the maxillary teeth while centric relation occlusal stops are recorded against the mandibular teeth with Delar wax in the cuspid areas and Aluwax in the molar areas.

Occlusal Splint Fabrication Procedure

Various materials and techniques exist for the fabrication of occlusal splints and the treatment of occlusal and temporomandibular joint disorders. We will outline a procedure for fabrication of an occlusal splint mounted in centric relation on a semiadjustable articulator. The occlusion of the appliance will be adjusted on the articulator to provide centric relation occlusal stops and anterior disclusion on the cuspid teeth with end point crossover on the central incisors. We have found this occlusal arrangement to provide a stable occlusion for many occlusal disorders, including bruxism and many temporomandibular joint disorders. The fabrication of an occlusal splint of this type can be easily adapted to many types of splints and materials.

The dental assistant:

* Disinfects alginate impressions
* Pours alginate impressions with a type III dental stone
* Trims models on a model trimmer
* Mounts the upper model on an articulator using facebow transfer with an incisal pin set to 0

The doctor will mount the lower model on the articulator, using the centric relation record with the incisal pin opened to approximate the thickness of the centric relation record (2–5 mm).

The dental assistant:

* Removes both models from articulator, fills in mounting voids with mounting plaster, and smooths with water. When dry, smooths models with a fine-grade sandpaper under the faucet to create a smooth, shiny appearance
* Returns both models to the articulator, verifies final incisal pin setting, and records in notes (Fig. 1-29)
* Opens incisal pin to achieve appropriate minimum thickness of 2 mm in the posterior regions
* Applies separating medium to the maxillary model and lets it air dry
* Places blue wax around the exterior of the maxillary model at the gingival level
* Applies two more coats of separating medium to the maxillary model and lets it air dry
* Mixes acrylic until the stickiness is gone
* Rolls acrylic out and places it on maxillary model surface

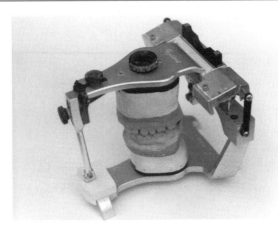

Figure 1-29. Accurately mounted models in centric relation occlusion with incisal pin setting at 0. The models are now ready for occlusal splint fabrication.

✳ Places wax paper between acrylic and mandibular model and closes articulator

✳ Checks that teeth are about 2 mm apart or closed enough until color shows through

✳ Lets acrylic set

✳ Trims occlusal splint and reverifies occlusion and excursions

✳ Polishes splint (Fig. 1-30)

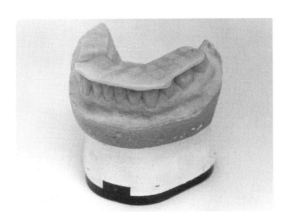

Figure 1-30. Finished occlusal splint on mandibular model ready for intraoral reline, adjustment, and delivery.

Occlusal Splint Reline and Delivery Procedure

Operatory Preparation

Barriers

Prior to seating the patient, the dental assistant will place the appropriate infection control barriers in the operatory. These include plastic covering for all surfaces that may become contaminated and that will not be disinfected with an aerosol spray following the procedure. Such surfaces may include

- overhead light handles and light switches
- operatory delivery systems
- plastic tubing for handpieces and suction

- nitrous oxide equipment
- x-ray heads
- doctor and assistant stools
- headrest on the dental chair

Personal protective equipment (eyewear, masks, and gloves) will be available and ready to use during the procedure for both the doctor and the dental assistant. Protective eyewear will also be provided for the patient.

Exam Tray (Fig. 1-31)

- ✓ instruments (mouth mirror, explorer, periodontal probe, cotton pliers)
- ✓ 2×2s
- ✓ cotton rolls
- ✓ high-volume evacuator
- ✓ saliva ejector

- ✓ air-water tip
- ✓ articulating paper on forceps
- ✓ cold cure or auto cure acrylic powder and monomer liquid
- ✓ hot water
- ✓ occlusal splint

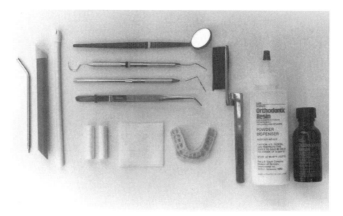

Figure 1-31. Standard tray setup for occlusal splint reline procedure. Included are articulating paper on forceps, cold cure acrylic, and occlusal splint.

After tray setup is complete, the dental assistant will set up the following:

✳ Handpieces: slow-speed with straight nose cone and acrylic bur

Seating Patient

The dental assistant:

✳ Greets the patient, places the bib, and discusses the appointment with the patient

Preparation

The dental assistant

✳ Tries in the fabricated splint and checks for rocking, bulkiness, fit, and bite

The doctor:

✳ Makes any necessary adjustments (e.g., grinding out splint for new fit or trimming bulk)

The dental assistant:

✳ Fills a green rubber bowl with hot water
✳ Mixes cold cure acrylic powder into a large rubber bowl with a few drops of monomer until a very runny consistency has been achieved
✳ Prepares inside of the splint with monomer and immediately pours the runny acrylic mixture into the splint
✳ Dips the splint into hot water for a few seconds to reduce the monomer taste and hands the splint to the doctor

The doctor:

✳ Seats the splint and removes the excess acrylic
✳ Has the patient bite into the splint for approximately 5 minutes and removes splint after the acrylic is set

The dental assistant:

✳ Trims all interproximal areas and smooths the splint with an acrylic bur
✳ Reseats the splint and with 2×2s and articulating paper on forceps, and records centric relation and lateral excursions for the doctor to adjust

Finish

The dental assistant:

✳ Reviews with the patient the benefits of occlusal splint therapy per the doctor's instructions and how to care for the splint

✳ Rinses the patient

✳ Finishes the chart entry and asks the doctor for the next appointment

✳ Removes the bib and walks the patient to the front desk

The dental assistant will now remove all the plastic barriers in the operatory, re-place them with new ones, and spray all contaminated surfaces with an OSHA-approved disinfectant to get the operatory ready for the next patient.

 N O T E
The authors suggest that users of this text review their current state infection control regulations and modify these procedures if necessary.

Occlusal Splint Adjustment Procedure

Operatory Preparation

Barriers

Prior to seating the patient, the dental assistant will place the appropriate infection control barriers in the operatory. These include plastic covering for all surfaces that may become contaminated and that will not be disinfected with an aerosol spray following the procedure. Such surfaces may include

- overhead light handles and light switches
- operatory delivery systems
- plastic tubing for handpieces and suction
- nitrous oxide equipment
- x-ray heads
- doctor and assistant stools
- headrest on the dental chair

Personal protective equipment (eyewear, masks, and gloves) will be available and ready to use during the procedure for both the doctor and the dental assistant. Protective eyewear will also be provided for the patient.

Exam Tray

- ✓ instruments (mouth mirror, explorer, periodontal probe, cotton pliers)
- ✓ 2×2s
- ✓ cotton rolls
- ✓ high-volume evacuator
- ✓ saliva ejector
- ✓ air-water tip
- ✓ articulating paper on forceps

After tray setup is complete, the dental assistant will set up the following:

∗ Handpieces: slow-speed with straight nose cone and acrylic bur

Seating Patient

The dental assistant:

∗ Greets the patient, places the bib, and discusses the appointment with the patient

Adjustment

The doctor:

∗ Has the patient try in the occlusal splint to check the fit; if there is any rocking or it does not seat, new impressions will be taken

✳ Checks lateral excursions with 2×2s and articulating paper on forceps

✳ Checks centric stops with 2×2s and articulating paper on forceps

✳ Removes heavy centric stops and balancing interferences using a slow-speed handpiece and acrylic bur

The dental assistant:

✳ Polishes the occlusal splint after all the adjustments have been made

Finish

The dental assistant:

✳ Reviews with the patient why he or she is wearing an occlusal splint and how to care for it

✳ Rinses the patient

✳ Finishes the chart entry and asks the doctor for the next appointment

✳ Removes the bib and walks the patient to the front desk

The dental assistant will now remove all the plastic barriers in the operatory, replace them with new ones, and spray all contaminated surfaces with an OSHA-approved disinfectant to get the operatory ready for the next patient.

NOTE

The authors suggest that users of this text review their current state infection control regulations and modify these procedures if necessary.

Study Questions

1. What four items are common to every tray setup?

2. What is the first thing that is discussed with the patient and recorded in the chart after the patient has been seated?

3. What is the first thing that is done after the doctor has entered the operatory during a new patient examination appointment?

4. Existing restorations are charted in _____ and recorded on the _____.

5. Tooth surfaces to be restored are charted in _____ and listed in the order to be treated on the _____.

6. What question do you ask the doctor before releasing the patient?

7. An appropriate bur for the high-speed handpiece to begin an amalgam procedure is _____; for the slow-speed handpiece it is _____.

8. Appropriate burs for the high-speed handpiece to begin a composite procedure are _____ or _____.

9. A dental dam is (optional or mandatory) for a root canal procedure.

10. A dental dam is prepared with _____ hole(s) for a root canal procedure.

11. _____ pliers are used to adjust removable partial denture framework.

12. The dental assistant explains and has the oral surgery patient sign the _____ form prior to the procedure and explains the _____ instructions to the patient following the procedure.

13. Maxillary universal forceps are #_____, while mandibular universal forceps are #_____.

Duties of the Dental Assistant

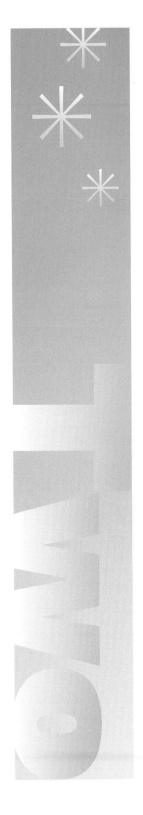

Objectives

The dental assistant plays a key role in delivering patient care in the contemporary dental office. Part of becoming a good team player is learning the skills and qualifications necessary to assist the doctor. Some of the following skills and qualifications you have already learned in preclinical courses, while others you will learn and master in the clinical setting. These include the following:

Sterilization and Infection Control

Seating, Releasing, and Discussion of the Procedure with the Patient

Radiographic Techniques

Taking Alginate Impressions

Boxing, Pouring, and Trimming Stone Models

Coronal Polish and Oral Hygiene Instruction

Pit and Fissure Sealant Application

Placement of Topical Anesthetic

Placement of the Dental Dam

Evacuation Technique: High-Volume and Saliva Ejector

Instrument Passing/Four-Handed Dentistry

Preparing the Tofflemire Retainer and Matrix

Polishing Amalgam

Shade Matching

Placement of Retraction Cord

Fabrication of Temporary Crowns (Vacuform Shell)

Mixing and Delivery of Cements

Measuring Endodontic Instruments

Administration/Scheduling

Operating Position/Ergonomics

There are many aspects and procedures of sterilization and infection control that are necessary and vital for the dental team to operate in a safe, noncontaminated environment. The authors acknowledge that codes and guidelines vary from state to state and recommend that the users of this book consult with their state department of health and/or the Department of Labor and Industries for specific information. We will provide an overview of the various aspects and the procedures we feel should be employed to obtain a safe working environment and form the minimum "backbone" of a more detailed, customized written plan that should be available in every dental office setting. Part of a safe working environment includes the OSHA standard requiring that the hepatitis B vaccination be made available to all employees with occupational exposure. We will start with a section on barriers for the operatory and setting up for a procedure; breakdown and cleaning up of the operatory following a procedure; cleaning, bagging, and sterilization of instruments and handpieces; preparing tray setups; and maintenance of operatories and sterilization areas.

Operatory Infection Control Barriers

Prior to seating the patient, the dental assistant will place appropriate infection control barriers in the operatory. These include plastic covering for all surfaces that may become contaminated and that will not be disinfected with an aerosol spray following the procedure. Such surfaces may include:

- overhead light handles and light switches
- operatory delivery systems
- plastic tubing for handpieces
- air-water syringe and suction tubing

- nitrous oxide equipment
- x-ray heads
- doctor and assistant stools
- headrest on the dental chair (Fig. 2-1)

Tray Setup

The tray setup shall include all the appropriate instruments for the procedure in a sealed bag or in a cartridge system that has been wrapped and sterilized by heat, steam, or chemical vapor. The contents may be opened and placed on the tray and then covered with a patient bib to prevent contamination. Bagged, sterilized handpieces are opened at the same time and are prerun with fiberoptics on.

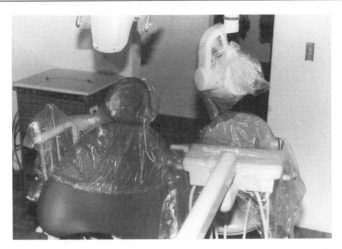

Figure 2-1. Plastic barriers are placed on all surfaces that may become contaminated during a procedure and that will not be disinfected following the procedure.

Personal Protection

Personal protective equipment will be available and ready to use during each procedure for the doctor, dental hygienist, and dental assistant. It should include the following:

- gowns
- eyewear
- masks
- gloves

Gowns. These should be fluid resistant, and should cover the employee's clothing and as much exposed skin as possible. If the garment becomes visibly soiled, it should be changed at once. Protective gowns should not be worn outside the clinical area, including staff lounges and the reception area. Contaminated gowns should be placed in a laundry bag identified by the international "Biohazard" symbol when soiled or at the end of each day, whichever comes first. This bag will then be picked up by a professional laundry service. If a staff member is designated to perform laundry services within the office, personal protective equipment must be worn when handling the contaminated laundry and a 1:100 bleach-to-water solution must be added to the hot water and laundry detergent in the washing machine. Following the washing cycle, the clean laundry must be machine dried prior to use. *Under no circumstances* is contaminated laundry to be removed from the office premises by any staff member.

Eyewear. Eyewear is to be worn by everyone involved in a clinical procedure, including the patient, and should have top and side extensions for maximum protection against splatter and flying debris. Protective eyewear should be cleaned and disinfected according to the manufacturer's instructions between patient visits.

Masks. Clear plastic face shields may be worn instead of protective eyewear when massive amounts of splatter are anticipated. Protective masks are worn over the nose and mouth and are discarded after each patient visit. These masks are to be worn with protective eyewear or face shields.

Gloves. These are to be worn after the hands have been thoroughly washed and dried and must be discarded following each patient visit. Vinal gloves should be available for latex-sensitive persons.

Postprocedure Sterilization

Surfaces. Following the procedure, the contaminated tray, instruments, and handpieces are taken to the sterilization area for cleaning and sterilization. The dental assistant then removes all plastic barriers in the operatory and replaces them with new ones. All contaminated surfaces are then disinfected using the following spray-wipe-spray technique:

- *Spray* all contaminated surfaces with an OSHA-approved disinfectant.
- *Wipe* surfaces with a paper towel to clean them.
- *Spray* surfaces again, leaving them wet for an additional *10 minutes* for disinfection.

Once the operatory has been prepared for the next patient, the dental assistant is ready to take care of the contaminated tray setup.

Instruments. The dental assistant should begin all procedures in the sterilization area by wearing heavy-duty rubber utility gloves and appropriate personal protective equipment. All instruments should be placed in the ultrasonic bath for at least *10 minutes* to loosen the debris. If the ultrasonic unit is unavailable, the instruments are placed in a holding tank with cleaning solution to keep the instruments and debris wet. When the 10-minute ultrasonic cycle has been completed, the ultrasonic tray is removed from the bath by the handles and the instruments are rinsed underwater. The ultrasonic tray is then inverted over a cotton towel that will be used to blot dry the instruments. Once dry, all instruments from the original tray setup should be bagged together using appropriate tape and bagging material with indicators for sterilization.

The following should be placed in a puncture-resistant sharps container marked with the international "Biohazard" label:

- anesthetic needles
- carpules
- scalpel blades

- burs
- suture needles
- broken instruments

Any blood-soaked gauze or cotton rolls should be placed in an impervious container labeled with the international "Biohazard" label or in the sharps container. Disposable materials including

- gloves
- masks
- wipes
- patient bibs
- surface covers

that are contaminated with body fluids should be handled carefully, with the above-mentioned utility gloves on, and discarded in sturdy, impervious plastic bags to minimize human contact.

Handpieces. Handpieces and bur blocks should be bagged separately. For most high-speed handpieces, following a procedure the handpiece should be lubricated and run for approximately *one minute* with the water on, then wiped clean. This is also recommended for flushing the water lines between patients. Again, the authors recommend the review of the specific manufacturer's instructions. At this point, the bags are ready to be put into the sterilization chamber for sterilization.

Sterilization Equipment

Many types of equipment for sterilization are available today; the most common types for many offices are the chemical vapor sterilizer and the steam cassette autoclave. It is important for both types to have good airflow throughout the chamber. This can be accomplished by following the manufacturer's instructions for usage and overfilling. Most dental bagging material and tapes have chemical indicators that change color when a certain temperature in the sterilization chamber has been reached. Although this may be a satisfactory method for determining batch-to-batch sterilization efficiency, it does not confirm that the appropriate pressure has been reached in the sterilization chamber. Since sterilization is a function of both temperature and pressure, all equipment used for the sterilization of instruments and handpieces should by monitored weekly with a spore test that is sent to an approved independent laboratory for analysis and a report. The reports must be kept on file as part of the documentation requirements of the exposure control program.

After the sterilization cycle is completed, the bagged instruments are placed unopened on a disinfected tray in the cabinet for a future appointment. Bagged handpieces and bur blocks are also placed unopened in the appropriate storage areas for future procedures. Many elaborate systems are used to identify instruments and trays for specific procedures. Instruments can be grouped with color-coded plastic bands, and many trays systems are color coded. Instruments from various tray setups should not be mixed during cleaning and bagging to avoid confusion and sorting before or after sterilization.

End-of-Day Procedures

At the end of each day, the dental assistant will run a cleaning solution through the suction tubes, flush the handpiece lines for 3 minutes, and check the traps in each operatory. The following solutions are to be changed as indicated:

- glutaraldehyde
- holding tank
- ultrasonic
- spray-wipe-spray disinfectant

Sharps containers are checked, disposed of, and changed as indicated. Autoclave chambers are inspected and cleaned as indicated. The following items should be disinfected following usage and prior to the end of the day:

- impressions
- laboratory handpieces and burs used on clinical prosthetic devices
- countertop areas in the operatories and the sterilization area

Seating, Releasing, and Discussing the Procedure with the Patient

Three important duties of the dental assistant for every procedure are: greeting and seating of the patient, discussing and reviewing of the procedure, and dismissing or walking the patient to the front desk. Since the dental assistant may have the first and/or the last contact with the patient before the patient leaves the office, it is critical that every effort be made to create a positive experience for the patient.

Greeting the Patient

When greeting the patient in the reception area:

- make eye contact
- address the patient with the appropriate title (Mr., Mrs., or Ms. and the last name)
- smile as you introduce yourself
- show the patient to the appropriate treatment room
- offer to hang up or show the patient where to place his or her hat, coat, purse, and so on

Preprocedure Conversation

Understanding that many patients may be apprehensive prior to dental procedures, making small talk or chatting with the patient prior to reviewing his or her health history will, in most cases, help to relax the patient. Patients who are reluctant to carry on a conversation with you may be offered a magazine to read while waiting for the doctor to begin the procedure.

After seating the patient, the dental assistant:

- places the bib
- discusses the procedure to be performed
- asks the patient if there are any questions

Again, eye contact with the patient is important here, and the patient should have your undivided attention. All questions should be answered to the best of your ability; if you are uncertain, refer the question to the doctor. Following any questions, the dental assistant then summons the doctor to begin the procedure.

Postprocedure Conversation

Following the completion of the procedure, the dental assistant:

- finishes the chart entry
- reviews any pertinent information about the procedure as instructed by the doctor
- reviews prescriptions or postoperative instructions that the doctor has written
- asks the patient if there are any questions before removing the bib

Dismissal of the Patient

The dental assistant now removes the bib and before leaving the operatory, gets the patient's hat, coat, purse, and so on as needed. Check to see if the patient needs another appointment before walking the patient to the front desk. Remember to smile and make eye contact. The patient will remember and will usually appreciate your effort to make the experience pleasant.

Radiographic Techniques

When taking dental radiographs, the dental assistant should take care to minimize the radiation exposure to the patient. This can be achieved through the use of the following equipment:

- lead apron with thyroid collar
- appropriate high-speed dental x-ray film
- appropriately calibrated x-ray equipment
- appropriate film holders and targets

An example of the RINN XCP system and the VIP system are shown below (Fig. 2-2A,B).

The authors recognize that many experienced dental assistants obtain excellent diagnostic radiographs with the use of bite tabs and no targeting equipment; however, for instructional purposes, we recommend the use of film holders and targeting equipment. The use of such equipment will assist the dental assistant in lining up the x-ray position indicator device with the film packet and the teeth and ultimately produce accurate diagnostic radiographs.

Preparation of Equipment

When taking dental radiographs, the switches on the control panel for exposure time, kilovoltage, and milliamperage should not be changed from the standard office settings unless instructed by the doctor. Plastic barriers should be placed

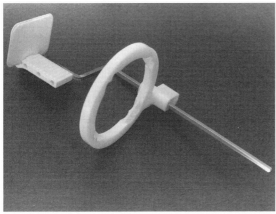
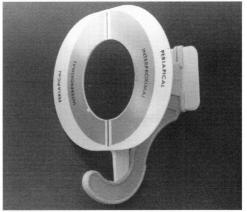

A   **B**

Figure 2-2. Example of (**A**) RINN XCP and (**B**) VIP radiographic equipment showing the corresponding film holders and targets.

over all equipment that may become contaminated during the procedure, including the x-ray position indicator device and control panel. The lead apron should not be touched with contaminated gloves and should be decontaminated after every appointment.

Paralleling Technique

With modern dental radiographic equipment, it is possible to consistently obtain excellent diagnostic radiographs using a paralleling technique. In using this technique for either bitewing or periapical radiographs, it is important to remember the following:

- the film packet and holder should be placed as parallel to the long axis of the teeth and as close to the teeth as possible
- the x-ray position indicator device should be in line perpendicular to the teeth and the film packet
- the patient should bite completely together on the film holder

The film packet should always be placed with the white side facing the operator or toward the x-ray position indicator device. If the tab on the film packet is facing the operator, a herringbone pattern from the lead will be produced on the developed radiograph.

When taking maxillary periapical radiographs, it is sometimes necessary to move the film packet and holder toward the middle of the palate while maintaining parallelism to the long axis of the teeth. Likewise, when taking mandibular periapical radiographs, it may be necessary to curve the border of the film packet to prevent impingement of the muscles on the floor of the mouth. This will prevent bending of the film packet and eventual distortion in the radiographs.

Taking Alginate Impressions

Taking accurate alginate impressions is one of the most important functions that the dental assistant will perform. These impressions will later be converted into the following:

- diagnostic study models that will be used by the doctor for analysis of occlusion
- fabrication of a vacuum-formed matrix for temporary crowns/bridges
- fabrication of custom acrylic impression trays
- fabrication of occlusal splints and bleaching trays
- opposing models for fixed and removable prosthodontic cases

When taking alginate impressions, the following anatomical details must be recorded:

- all visible tooth surfaces, including buccal, lingual, and occlusal surfaces
- extension into and through the buccal vestibule
- maxillary tuberosity for maxillary impressions
- retromolar pad for mandibular impressions

The impressions should be centered over the incisor teeth and free of voids, tears, or perforations.

Choosing an Impression Tray

Choosing the appropriate impression tray for the patient is the first step in recording an accurate impression. Many acceptable impression trays are available, and the dental assistant should be familiar with the tray retention style prior to patient use. The authors recommend the use of *stock metal trays without perforations* for simplicity of use and cleanup. If the patient already has a set of study models, the dental assistant can choose a tray of the appropriate size prior to the procedure. If the dental assistant is taking impressions on a patient for the first time, he or she should try in trays to find a size that is comfortable for the patient and has adequate extensions to record the required anatomical structures listed above. Prior to taking the impression, it is sometimes necessary to add utility wax to the border of the impression tray to extend the length and/or depth of the tray.

Preparing the Alginate

After the impression tray has been selected and, if necessary, adapted with utility wax, the dental assistant is ready to begin mixing the alginate material. There are many brands of alginate impression material, and most are available in premixed packages or in bulk containers. Again, it is important to be familiar with the manufacturer's instructions for the product you are using prior to patient use. In general, maxillary impressions require *three* scoops of powdered alginate material and *three* measures of water; mandibular impressions require *two* scoops of powdered alginate material and *two* measures of water. When mixing, *always* add alginate to the water (room temperature or slightly cooler) in a flexible rubber bowl.

Mixing the Alginate

Begin mixing by using a wide-blade metal spatula and incorporate the alginate powder with the water. After several seconds, mix the alginate, using a forceful spatulation or beating against the sides of the mixing bowl, squeezing the alginate between the spatula and the bowl (Fig. 2-3). A smooth, creamy, homogeneous mixture should be obtained within 30–45 seconds.

The impression tray is then loaded with the alginate material and is ready for placement. Alginate may be wiped on the occlusal surfaces of the teeth and injected into the vestibule with a large plastic syringe prior to tray placement, but this is not necessary to record accurate impressions.

It is helpful to record mandibular impressions first to get the patient accustomed to the procedure before the possibility of activating the gag reflex on maxillary impressions.

On maxillary impressions, take care to load the posterior section of the tray with only enough material to record the required anatomical structures, including

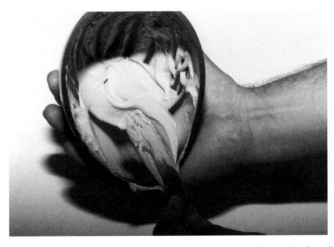

Figure 2-3. Spatulation of alginate impression material between the mixing bowl and the spatula.

the hard palate. This can be accomplished by feathering the alginate material with the spatula toward the posterior border of the tray, leaving only 3–4 mm of material at the border of the tray. This is important to avoid activating the patient's gag reflex while still having enough material to record several millimeters of the soft palate.

Mandibular Impressions

For mandibular impressions, the dental assistant stands *in front* of the patient and gently retracts the patient's right cheek with the left index finger while rotating the loaded impression tray clockwise into position against the left cheek. This will allow plenty of room for insertion and minimize unwanted alginate transfer to the patient's face.

After the tray has been positioned and the handle centered over the incisor teeth, the dental assistant will hold the tray in place using the index fingers on top of the tray, while the thumbs are positioned gently under the patient's chin. This will help to maintain even finger pressure and keep the tray level over the teeth.

At this point, check to be sure that the tray is not impinging on the lips or cheeks, and have the patient lift the tongue and then let the tongue fall to the floor of the mouth.

Maxillary Impressions

For maxillary impressions, the dental assistant stands *behind* the patient and gently retracts the patient's left cheek with the left index finger while rotating the loaded impression tray counterclockwise into position against the right cheek.

After the tray has been positioned and the handle centered over the incisor teeth, the dental assistant holds the tray in place using the index and middle fingers under the tray, keeping even pressure from left to right. Again, the dental assistant must check to be sure that the tray is not impinging on the patient's lips or cheeks.

Setting Time of the Impression

While the impression material is setting, the patient can be holding the mixing bowl for the dental assistant to evaluate the setting time. Although not a necessary step, this may be helpful for familiarization of the impression material and will involve the patient in the procedure.

When the impression material is set, the dental assistant breaks the seal by running the index finger between the border of the impression and the cheek. For *mandibular* impressions the dental assistant should stand *in front* of the patient.

The thumb should be placed under the handle and the tray removed with a firm lifting motion, keeping at least two fingers on top of the tray to protect the maxillary teeth. For *maxillary* impressions the dental assistant should stand *behind* the patient. The thumb should be placed on top of the handle and the tray removed with a firm downward motion, keeping at least two fingers under the tray to protect the mandibular teeth.

Once the impressions have been removed and evaluated for accuracy, they are disinfected and prepared for pouring with the appropriate dental stone.

Boxing, Pouring, and Trimming Study Casts

Following appropriate disinfection of alginate impressions, the dental assistant is ready to create diagnostic study casts. Attention to detail when boxing the impression, measuring and mixing the dental stone, and pouring the dental stone into the model will result in accurate study casts that will be trimmed and stored as part of the patient's permanent records.

Preparation of the Completed Impression

After the alginate impression has been disinfected, all excess material beyond the depth of the vestibule should be removed from the border of the tray. This will aid in the final trimming of the model.

Prior to boxing the mandibular impression, a tongue space is added to the impression. This is created by inverting the impression on a glass slab and mixing one unit of alginate material to be spread between the dentition in the lingual space.

Boxing the Impression

Boxing of the impression may be done with either a roll of utility wax or duct tape. On a glass slab, wrap the duct tape around the circumference of the impression, forming a seal to the border of the impression (Fig. 2-4).

Following the manufacturer's instructions, incorporate the appropriate amount

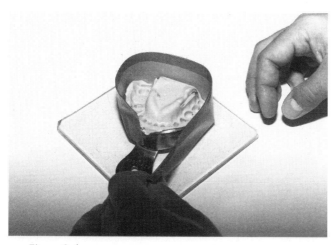

Figure 2-4. Boxing an alginate impression with duct tape.

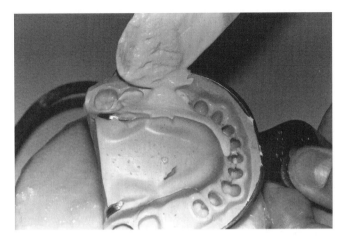

Figure 2-5. Pouring the alginate impression with dental stone.

of water in the dental stone in a flexible rubber mixing bowl using a wide-bladed metal spatula.

Finish mixing by placing the bowl on a mechanical vibrator to eliminate bubbles in the stone. In some cases, the doctor will recommend the use of a sealed plastic bowl and a vacuum mixer to prepare a type IV dental die stone mixture.

Pouring the Impression

Begin pouring the impression by tilting it at an angle on the mechanical vibrator and letting the dental stone run down from the blade of the spatula into the impression (Fig. 2-5).

Continue to vibrate the dental stone into the impression until all tooth surfaces have been covered and no bubbles are present.

At this point, place the impression on the glass slab and finish pouring the dental stone into the boxed impression to the desired level. If the dental assistant is using a duct tape border, filling the impression to the top of the tape will usually result in adequate thickness for the base of the study cast.

Once the pouring of the impression has been completed, allow the dental stone to set or harden for at least 45 minutes.

Separation, Cleanup, and Trimming of the Models

Once the dental stone has hardened, the dental assistant uses a laboratory knife to separate the border of the impression from the stone model.

The impression tray is then lifted up from the model, being careful not to fracture the teeth on the model.

Once the tray has been removed from the model, any imperfections or nerds are removed with a sharp Cleoid-Discoid or Hollenback carving instrument under magnification.

The study casts are then trimmed to the appropriate geometric dimensions, as instructed by the doctor. Unmounted orthodontic study casts are usually sharply trimmed to exact patterns and buffed to a glossy surface. This is not necessary for mounting study casts on an articulator, nor is it appropriate for removable prosthodontic models in which the entire depth of the vestibule is required to fabricate the prosthetic device.

A coronal polish is generally performed following scaling and/or root planing by the doctor or the hygienist and is one duty the dental assistant may be required to perform daily on children and some adult patients. It also forms the main part of the child and adult recall or checkup appointment, which also includes:

- examination by the doctor
- oral hygiene instruction
- scaling and root planing (if necessary)
- topical fluoride administration

In many offices, the dental assistant will perform the coronal polish only on children during the recall appointment, while the doctor or hygienist performs this procedure on adult patients.

Oral Hygiene Instruction

In the child recall appointment, the dental assistant asks the child to demonstrate his or her brushing and flossing technique. Tips and instructions to improve the child's technique may be given at this time, along with praise for areas that were cleaned well.

The child then finishes brushing to the best of his or her ability. The dental assistant will now use a disclosing solution or disclosing tablets to temporarily color the plaque red to make it visible.

Using a large hand mirror, the child then evaluates, with help from the dental assistant, the quality of the brushing technique. Again, tips and instructions are critical at this point while the child can see the red areas that were missed while brushing. When thorough oral hygiene instructions have been completed, the teeth may be polished.

The Coronal Polish

Using a slow-speed handpiece with prophy angle and rubber cup, the teeth are polished with prophy paste in a cervical-to-incisal direction. The prophy cup should reach all visible surfaces of the clinical crowns for all teeth present. It is important to polish to the gum line since this is a common area for plaque accumulation (Fig. 2-6). In areas where the patient is having difficulty reaching with the brush or where there is excess plaque or stain, a bristle brush may be used.

During the procedure, the child should use the hand mirror to watch as plaque and stain are removed from the teeth.

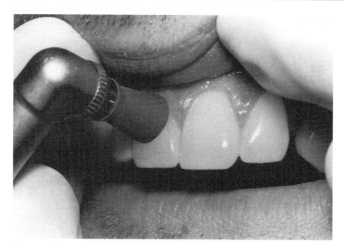

Figure 2-6. Prophy cup polishing technique at the gingival surface.

The disclosing solution or tablets can also be used by the dental assistant as an indicator to evaluate the thoroughness of the polish. No disclosing solution should remain at the end of the coronal polish. In addition, the dental assistant may ask the child to hold the saliva ejector. This is a good way to achieve active participation during the procedure. The dental assistant finishes the cleaning by flossing through all proximal contacts.

Topical Fluoride Administration

Following the coronal polish, topical fluoride is administered. Many types and brands of fluoride are available today, ranging from foam to gels administered in disposable trays, fluoride rinses, and topical fluoride that is painted on the teeth with cotton swabs or a toothbrush. A saliva ejector should be used with the fluoride trays and the paint-on fluoride to minimize ingestion. After examination by the doctor, the dental assistant or the doctor reviews the home care instructions with the child and parent and gives the child a package of home care aides, including a toothbrush, floss, and disclosing tablets.

Pit and Fissure Sealant Application

Pit and fissure sealants have been one of the most effective preventive procedures in fighting dental caries since the application of topical fluoride. The procedure can be done quickly and is noninvasive. However, pit and fissure sealants are technique sensitive and require attention to detail at every step. It is imperative that the doctor has recently examined the teeth to be sealed to ensure that no caries are present on either the occlusal or proximal surfaces.

The most commonly sealed teeth in children are the *first and second permanent molars*. Because of the eruption sequence, sealants are usually done in two phases.

- The first phase occurs at approximately *6* years of age or when the *first* permanent molars have fully erupted.
- The second phase occurs at approximately *12* years of age or when the *second* permanent molars have fully erupted.

There is no age limit for sealing teeth; in fact, sealants for adult patients may be indicated if there is a sudden change of health that may increase the susceptibility to caries. The premolar teeth generally are not sealed due to their more shallow or less well defined occlusal anatomy and their correspondingly decreased susceptibility to caries.

Sealant Procedure

Before starting the procedure, the teeth to be sealed are cleaned of all plaque and debris with peroxide and a slow-speed handpiece with a prophy cup and/or brush. At this point, it is critical that the teeth to be sealed remain in a dry environment, and it is recommended that the teeth be sealed one at a time (Fig. 2-7). This can be accomplished with the use of a dental dam or cotton rolls and/or dry-aid isolation.

Once the tooth has been isolated, the occlusal surface is etched with a 37–40% phosphoric acid solution or gel for 10 to 30 seconds based on the manufacturer's instructions (Fig. 2-8).

The tooth is then rinsed with water for approximately 30 seconds and dried. The occlusal surface should now have a chalky or frosty white appearance and should remain completely dry while the sealant material is applied with a small brush or explorer (Fig. 2-9).

If the tooth is contaminated with saliva prior to sealant placement, it should be re-etched and dried for the full amount of time recommended. Only enough

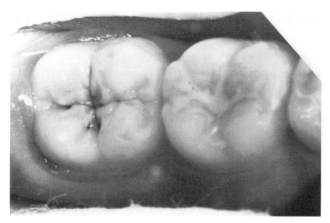

Figure 2-7. Tooth #31 prepared to receive occlusal sealant; tooth #30 has previously been sealed.

sealant material is applied to fill in the pits and grooves so as not to alter the patient's occlusion.

The sealant material is then light cured for 30 to 60 seconds, depending on the manufacturer's instructions (Fig. 2-10).

The dental assistant then checks the occlusion with articulating paper on forceps and the retention of the sealant with an explorer. When all sealants have been finished, the doctor evaluates the retention and adjusts the occlusion as necessary (Fig. 2-11).

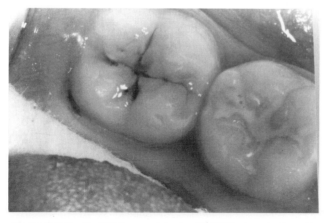

Figure 2-8. Tooth #31 being etched with 37% phosphoric acid.

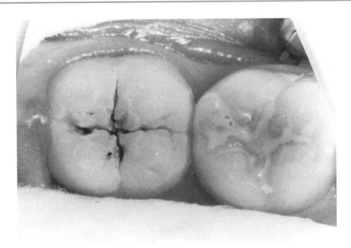

Figure 2-9. Tooth #31 with etched enamel surface ready for placement of sealant material.

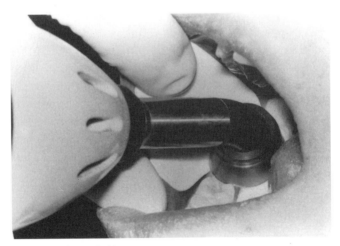

Figure 2-10. Light-curing the sealant material.

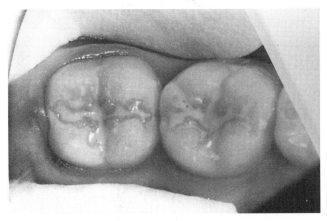

Figure 2-11. Completed occlusal sealants.

Placement of Topical Anesthetic

The dental assistant's role in preparing a patient for an operative procedure begins with the correct placement of topical anesthetic. The surface tissues will then be numb enough to significantly decrease the pain associated with the initial needle penetration during the injection. The following steps are important to achieve adequate topical anesthesia.

Prior to placement, the area which will receive the topical anesthetic should be *dried with a 2×2 gauze pad.* This will help facilitate absorption of the anesthetic across the mucous membrane and prevent unwanted dilution of the anesthetic during placement. Whether in liquid or ointment form, the anesthetic should be placed on the end of a cotton-tipped applicator (Q-tip), which will then be placed in the correct area of the mouth for *1–2 minutes* but no longer.

Maxillary Placement

Anesthesia for maxillary teeth is usually accomplished by buccal infiltration near the apex of the tooth (or teeth) to be restored. Therefore, the cotton tip with topical anesthetic is placed in the buccal vestibule above the appropriate tooth (teeth) for 1–2 minutes (Fig. 2-12).

Mandibular Placement

Anesthesia for mandibular teeth is accomplished by blocking the inferior alveolar nerve. Topical anesthetic is placed between the coronoid notch and pterygomandibular raphe approximately 1 cm above the occlusal plane (Fig. 2-13).

If only the mental branch of the inferior alveolar nerve is to be blocked, topical anesthetic is placed between the premolars at the depth of the buccal vestibule. For buccal anesthesia, the long buccal nerve is blocked and topical anesthetic is placed alongside the molars at the depth of the buccal vestibule.

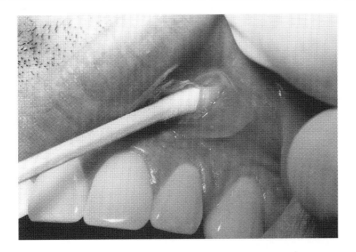

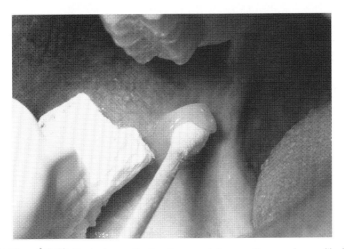

Figures 2-12 and 2-13. Topical anesthetic placement for maxillary and mandibular teeth.

Placement of the Dental Dam

After adequate local anesthesia has been obtained, the dental assistant isolates the operating field by placing the dental dam. A well-placed dental dam is one of the most effective barriers used in dentistry and should be placed only on teeth that are free of plaque and debris. This will help to prevent slippage of the clamp and subsequent damage to gingival tissues. The dental dam:

- isolates the operating field for the dental team
- protects the patient's oral tissues from high-speed instrumentation and suspended debris such as tooth fragments and restorative materials

Dental Dam Materials

Dam material. The dental dam material comes in a wide variety of sizes, colors, and thicknesses. The most common size is a 6 × 6-inch square for the permanent dentition and a 5 × 5-inch square for the primary dentition. Color and thickness are chosen by the operator based on the strength and feel of the material and the desired background color of the operating field.

Frames. Dental dam frames are available in metal or plastic. The latter is used most commonly during endodontic procedures.

Napkins. Dental dam napkins, which are placed between the patient's face and dam material, along with lubricants such as petroleum jelly placed on the lips, can be used to enhance patient comfort while wearing the dental dam.

Selection of the Operating Field and Clamp

Prior to placing the dental dam, the dental assistant evaluates the area to be isolated and the tooth on which the clamp will be placed. The dental dam is to be placed at least one tooth *distal* to the tooth being restored, if possible, and extended to the midline or the opposite cuspid tooth, depending on the doctor's preference.

For root canal treatment, only the tooth involved is clamped and isolated.

For pediatric applications, the dental dam is prepared by punching *three* holes in a row and placing the clamp on the most distal tooth.

If the tooth has an average or long clinical crown, a clamp with flat jaws may be used. If the tooth has a short clinical crown, a clamp with curved jaws that will engage below the height of the tooth contour may be used.

In some cases, a special clamp is needed for gingival retraction of the facial

Maxillary arch

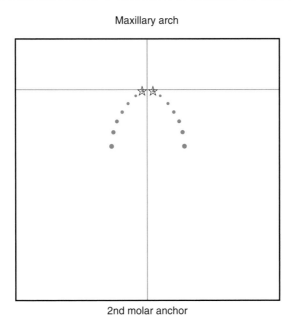

2nd molar anchor

Mandibular arch

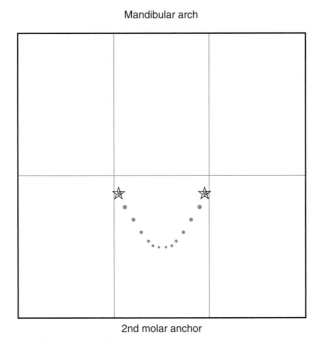

2nd molar anchor

Figures 2-14 and 2-15. Maxillary and mandibular arch dental dam templates.

surfaces of anterior teeth. Ferrier 212, 9, or W9 clamps work well under these circumstances and can be stabilized with red stick compound or red utility wax.

Placement of the Dental Dam

Once the appropriate clamp is selected, the dental dam is punched using the templates shown (Figs. 2-14, 2-15).

A piece of dental floss is tied to the clamp through the hole in the wing or jaw of the clamp and then looped around the bow as a precautionary measure.

The clamp is then placed through the rubber dam and on the most distal tooth of isolation. For the clamp to be secure, all four prongs must firmly engage the tooth.

Once the clamp is secured:

1. the dam material is stretched over the teeth
2. the frame is placed
3. the dental dam is flossed through the proximal contacts

The septa of the dental dam are then inverted using air and a blunt-ended instrument. A stabilizing cord, a piece of dental floss, or another clamp may be used to stabilize the end of the dam opposite the clamp if necessary.

The teeth are then rinsed and dried for the operative procedures to be performed.

Removal of the Dental Dam

When removing the dental dam, each septum should be cut before removing the clamp and frame. Following removal of the dental dam, the material should be inspected to ensure that there are no missing pieces. Any remaining pieces left in the patient's mouth can be removed with dental floss.

Evacuation Technique: High-Volume and Saliva Ejector

Mastering the evacuation of oral fluids and aerosol spray is one of the most challenging and frustrating aspects of dental assisting. Therefore, it is of great importance that the dental assistant develop the skills necessary to provide adequate evacuation as early in the formal training as possible. Successful evacuation technique can be developed through the use of a saliva ejector and/or high-volume evacuator (HVE).

Saliva Ejector

When the patient does not have dental dam isolation, it may be helpful for the learning dental assistant to use the saliva ejector as the primary source of evacuation unless the doctor is removing large amounts of tooth structure and/or restorative materials.

High-Volume Evacuator

When the dental assistant becomes more proficient and confident in the use of the more powerful HVE, the increased suction and retraction capabilities will be significant. The HVE should be used whenever possible for the above-mentioned reasons; however, it is important for the dental assistant to develop the skill necessary to operate the HVE without compromising the patient's comfort.

Hand Positions

After proper application of the rubber dam, the doctor and the dental assistant are ready to perform dentistry in an orderly and efficient manner. The two main hand positions for holding the HVE are:

- reverse palm-thumb grasp (Fig. 2-16A)
- modified pen grasp (Fig. 2-16B)

The authors prefer the palm-thumb grasp for the learning dental assistant because it offers greater control and retraction capability. The dental assistant should enter the patient's mouth first, attempting to place the suction tip parallel or slightly posterior to the tooth being prepared. It is absolutely necessary that the tip be placed *parallel* to the tooth, especially if a dental dam is not used.

Operating Position

When working from the *left* side of the patient's chair, the dental assistant places the HVE suction tip parallel to the buccal surfaces of the left maxillary and mandibular molars and lingual to the right maxillary and mandibular molars (Fig. 2-17).

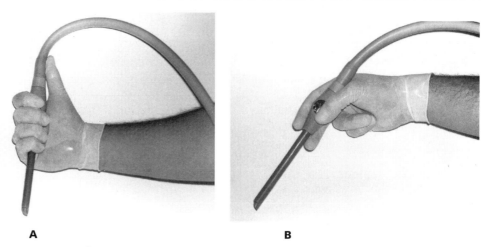

A   **B**

Figure 2-16. (**A**) Reverse palm-thumb grasp and (**B**) modified pen grasp for HVE suction tip.

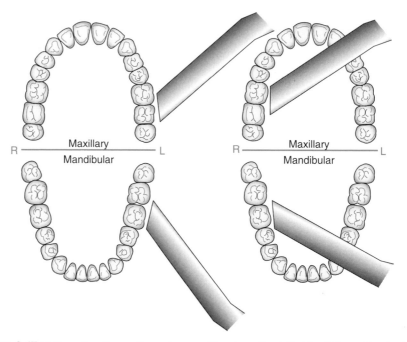

Figure 2-17. HVE suction tip position when working from the left side of the patient's chair.

When working from the *right* side of the patient's chair, the dental assistant places the HVE suction tip parallel to the lingual surfaces of the left maxillary and mandibular molars and buccal to the right maxillary and mandibular molars.

When working in the *anterior sextant* from either side of the patient's chair, the HVE suction tip should be placed parallel to the lingual surface of the tooth when the doctor is making the preparation from the facial surface and parallel to the facial surface of the tooth when the doctor is making the preparation from the lingual surface.

The proper transfer or passing of dental instruments is another skill that the dental assistant should master as quickly as possible. When this is accomplished, the operating efficiency between the doctor and the dental assistant improves and the time needed to complete many procedures decreases. The three most common ways to hold dental instruments are:

- pen grasp
- palm grasp
- reverse pen grasp

During most procedures, the dental assistant and doctor will use the *pen grasp* to hold hand instruments such as excavators, condensers, and carving instruments. The *palm grasp* is used to handle many oral surgery instruments and dental dam forceps, and the *reverse pen grasp* is used to hold a slow-speed handpiece equipped with a prophy angle.

When passing instruments to the doctor, the dental assistant should always pass them in such a way that the doctor does not have to:

- reach for an instrument
- look up from the procedure
- change the position or direction of the instrument

When assisting a *right*-handed doctor, the dental assistant will hold the HVE with the *right* hand while using the left hand to pass instruments or materials, operate the air-water syringe, and provide retraction of soft tissues. The reverse is true when assisting a left-handed doctor.

Figure 2-18A–E is helpful in understanding single-handed instrument transfer.

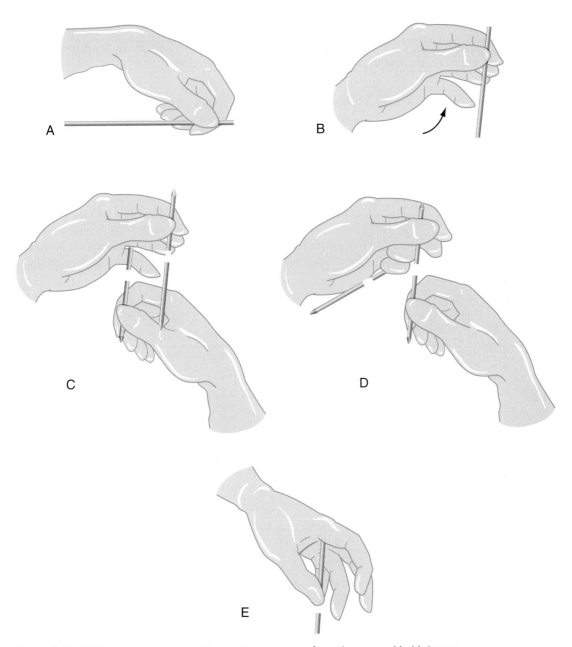

Figure 2-18. (**A**) The dental assistant picks up the instrument from the tray and holds it opposite the end to be used. (**B**) The new instrument is held with the thumb, and the index and third fingers are ready for passing. The little finger is extended to receive the used instrument. (**C**) The new instrument is aligned with the used instrument in the doctor's hand. (**D**) The doctor receives the new instrument with the nib in position to use while the dental assistant palms the used instrument after receiving it. (**E**) The thumb is used to rotate the used instrument into position for placement on the tray or to pass back to the doctor to reuse. (Modified with permission from Torres HO and Ehrlich A: *Modern Dental Assisting,* 4th ed., W.B. Saunders, Philadelphia, 1990.)

Preparing the Tofflemire Retainer and Matrix

The Tofflemire retainer and matrix band is one of the most popular items used in restorative dentistry to re-create interproximal surfaces and contacts. The Tofflemire matrices come in three sizes:

- universal
- molar
- premolar

The latter two sizes have two contoured loops and are sometimes referred to as "MOD bands." When laid on a flat surface, matrices of all three sizes are V-shaped and maintain this form even when viewed from the side as the ends are looped together prior to placement in the retainer (Fig. 2-19).

Assembling the Matrix and Retainer

The following three steps should be followed when assembling the Tofflemire matrix and retainer:

1. The Tofflemire retainer must always rest against the buccal surface of the teeth, whether maxillary or mandibular, unless instructed otherwise.
2. When the ends of the matrix are looped together and placed in the Tofflemire retainer, an MOD band or a straight band will form a V when viewed from the side. The apex of this V must always point toward the gin-

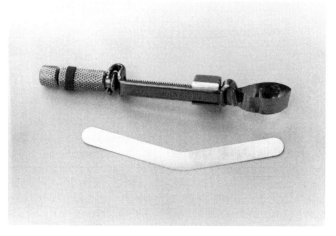

Figure 2-19. Flat and looped matrix band forming a V shape.

giva (vestibule), never toward the occlusal surface. (The occlusal surface of the matrix will have a greater circumference than the gingival surface.)

3. The opening of the slot on the Tofflemire retainer must also always point toward the gingiva (vestibule) for ease of removal. The matrix band may exit the retainer either straight through the slot or to the side, depending on the doctor's preference.

Placing the Matrix and Retainer over the Teeth

Once the Tofflemire retainer and matrix has been assembled, it is ready to be placed over the tooth to receive the restorative material. When placing the retainer with matrix over the tooth, the following must be done:

- All margins of the preparation must be enclosed within the contours of the matrix.
- The retainer is tightened to prevent the expression of restorative material into the gingival sulcus.
- When the matrix is tight, cotton pliers are used to place a wedge below the gingival margin with the flat end toward the gingival surface.
- Check to ensure that the proximal contact area is still intact, and use a ball burnisher to broaden the contact area.

After the restoration has been placed, the wedge is removed and the knob on the retainer is loosened. The doctor will then remove the retainer and matrix and finish contouring the restoration.

Polishing Amalgam

Although not required in contemporary dentistry, the authors still feel there is value in the polishing of dental amalgam. Many studies show that a well-polished amalgam increases the marginal seal and longevity of the filling and decreases the surface area available for plaque retention.

Amalgam should be polished no sooner than *24* hours following initial placement. This may be done as part of the recall or maintenance visits. A dental dam can be passively placed to enable the dental assistant to operate in a dry environment without worrying about retraction of the cheek and tongue.

Instruments

- examination tray with explorer
- mouth mirror
- articulating paper on forceps
- air-water syringe tip and HVE suction tip
- slow-speed handpiece with contra-angle and either a friction or latch-type head

Burs

- green stone or multibladed carbide finishing bur
- rubber abrasive points (brown, green, and super-green)
- mandrel with finishing discs
- prophy cup with fine pumice and powder abrasives

Polishing Sequence

The sequence for polishing amalgam is as follows:

1. The dental assistant checks the occlusion with 2×2s and articulating paper on forceps.
2. The doctor then corrects any gross discrepancies in occlusion or overhangs as necessary.
3. The dental assistant places a dental dam and begins polishing the margins of the restoration with a green stone or carbide finishing bur, always moving the bur in the direction from the restoration to the tooth.
4. The dental assistant polishes the margins with the brown, green, and super-green rubber abrasive points and the remainder of the restoration hold-

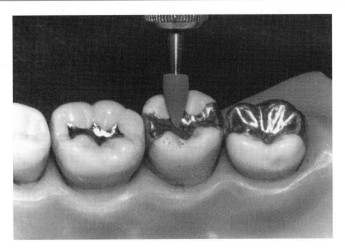

Figure 2-20. Polishing amalgam restoration with rubber abrasive point in a slow-speed handpiece with the tip pointed toward the central groove of the tooth.

ing the handpiece at a 45° angle toward the central groove of the tooth (Fig. 2-20).

5. The dental assistant polishes the occlusal surfaces with a prophy angle and cup with a tin-oxide powder at high speed and light pressure. Proximal surface margins may be polished with the abrasive powders or finishing discs; however, great care should be taken not to enter the interproximal contact area.

When finished, the margins should be nearly undetectable to an explorer and the occlusal surface should glisten.

Shade matching for the dental assistant is an important skill that takes time to develop, but when done well it will help the doctor to consistently predict esthetic outcomes. The following clinical procedures require shade matching:

- composites
- veneers
- crowns
- bridges
- dentures

When learning to match the color or shade of dental materials to tooth structure, an understanding of the three parameters of color is useful. They are hue, value, and chroma.

Hue. Hue, or the dominant wavelength of a color, is what we perceive as the visible color or shade, such as red, green, blue, or violet.

Value. Value is a measure of the lightness or darkness of a color and ranges from white (highest value) to black (lowest value).

Chroma. Chroma is the amount of saturation or intensity of a color.

VITA Shade Guide

All three parameters are important when considering the color of an object. One of the most popular systems for color determination of dental materials is the *VITA* shade guide (Fig. 2-21). In this system, four dominant colors, or hues, are repre-

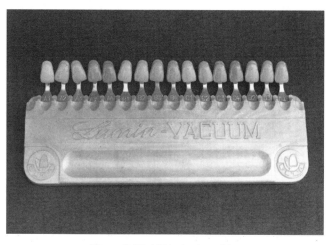

Figure 2-21. VITA shade guide.

sented. The A range has an orange hue, the B range has a yellow hue, and the C and D ranges have a gray hue. Within the A, B, C, and D ranges, colors become more saturated or intense as the numbers of the shade tab increase.

At the same time that the numbers of the shade tabs are increasing, the value of the color is decreasing. For example, the shade A2 has a higher value and less saturation or chroma than shade A4.

Color Evaluation Time and Conditions

When evaluating the color of teeth, the best time to determine the shade is when the patient first sits down in the chair. At this point, the teeth have not yet become dehydrated, which inevitably happens after cotton rolls or the dental dam has been placed. When teeth become dehydrated or desiccated, they usually turn one to two shades lighter. If the shade is chosen at this point, the esthetic outcome will be unsatisfactory when the teeth rehydrate. If possible, the shade should be determined in natural light by taking the patient to the window or even outside. If this is not possible, turn the overhead light *off* before determining the shade.

Composite

When anterior composite restorations are planned for the patient considering vital tooth bleaching, it is strongly recommended that the bleaching process be completed *prior* to placement of the composite restorations. This is because the composite materials and tooth structure change color at very different rates and some materials change color only slightly when exposed to bleaching solutions. Most of the composite materials available today blend very well with natural tooth structure; some manufacturers even claim that they exhibit a chameleon effect. Different shades may be used on the same tooth to reproduce natural changes in intensity from the gingival third of the tooth toward the incisal or occlusal surface. Also, the amount of tooth structure removed, as in a Class III or IV preparation, will determine if the doctor wants a more opaque core material to be veneered with a translucent material for the incisal edge. Many esthetic outcomes are possible, and the dental assistant should be familiar with all the composite materials in the office.

Prosthodontics

Many of the principles used for shade determination of composite materials can also be applied to fixed and removable prosthodontic procedures. When determining the shade for full-coverage preparations, a *35mm picture* with a VITA shade tab placed next to the tooth will give the laboratory technician the most accurate visual information regarding value, contour of adjacent teeth, and surface characteristics next to seeing the patient in person. Even after the fabrication of porcelain-bonded veneers and all porcelain crowns, the final color characteristics can be altered or adjusted through the use of colored cements and try-in pastes.

Finally, denture teeth may be matched to existing teeth, pictures of what the patient's teeth formerly looked like, and/or the patient's wishes. The shade and contour of the teeth will be chosen, and the patient should have an active role in the decision-making process.

Placement of Retraction Cord

The placement of gingival retraction cord for crown and bridge procedures is one of the most critical and potentially most invasive procedures required of the dental assistant. Extreme attention to detail is necessary to prevent tearing the gingival attachment while creating a hemorrhage-free gingival sulcus. When done well, impression taking will become routine and predictable for the doctor, the dental assistant, and the patient.

Many types of gingival retraction cord, packing instruments, and hemostatic agents are available today. This section describes a *double-pack technique* using braided retraction cord of different sizes and a blunt-ended packing instrument such as a plastic instrument or a blunted half-Hollenback.

Double-Pack Technique

- The smaller first cord protects the gingival attachment and biologic width while the tooth is prepared and serves as a guide or marker for the finish line of the preparation. It is not removed until the temporary crown has been cemented.
- The second, larger cord is placed after the tooth preparation has been completed, just before the impression is taken, and provides retraction or deflection of the gingival tissues.

In this technique, the first cord remains in the sulcus during the entire procedure. Its presence during impression taking promotes hemostasis and dramatically reduces the seepage of crevicular fluid.

Preparation of the Retraction Cord

Prior to placement, the dental assistant cuts the retraction cords to the approximate size and has the hemostatic agent ready. As a general rule when cutting retraction cord, the circumference of the little finger is used as a measurement for anterior teeth and premolars, and the circumference of the index finger is used as a measurement for molars. A cord that is slightly too long is always better than a cord that is too short.

Placement of the Retraction Cord

Once the interproximal contacts have been cleared, the initial cord (#00 or #0) is made into a loop and placed into the sulcus. When the first end of the cord has been placed, the remainder of the cord is tucked into the sulcus by gently rolling

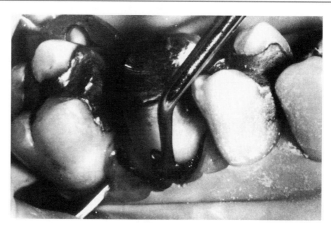

Figure 2-22. Placing gingival retraction cord.

the cord from the finish line on the tooth into the sulcus with the cord-packing instrument (Fig. 2-22). The tip of the instrument should always be directed toward and moving away from the cord that has already been placed. When the first cord is placed, the two ends should meet in a *butt-joint*. Sometimes it is necessary to trim the cord end prior to the final placement to meet in the butt-joint. A gap between the two ends is unacceptable since crevicular fluid can seep here.

When the tooth preparation has been completed, the second cord (#1 or #2) is placed in a similar manner, with the following exceptions: the cord is started in a different location to prevent dislodging the ends of the first cord, and a small tag of excess cord is left floating after the loop has been completed to alert the doctor to the cord end. Hemostatic agents may be used, if desired, on either cord.

When taking the impression, the doctor will remove the second cord, express the impression material around the tooth, and then place the impression tray. After the temporary crown has been fabricated and cemented, the dental assistant removes the first cord, leaving behind a clean, undamaged gingival sulcus.

Fabrication of Temporary Crowns (Vacuform Shell)

There are many satisfactory temporary crowns and crown fabricative methods, including the following:

- custom acrylic crown from a vacuform matrix coping
- preformed polycarbonate or metal crowns lined with acrylic

We will outline a method using a vacuform matrix taken from the preprepared tooth and cold cure acrylic. Properly fabricated temporary crowns replace existing tooth morphology and contour, hold the tooth in a static position by restoring interproximal contacts and occlusion, and reduce sensitivity until the patient receives the permanent restoration.

In the following order, the dental assistant will:

1. Prepare a quadrant vacuform matrix from a stone model of the patient's mouth prior to tooth preparation (Fig. 2-23).
2. Try in the vacuform matrix for fit and landmarks after the tooth has been prepared.
3. Lubricate the tooth with petroleum jelly.
4. Mix monomer and acrylic powder in a rubber cup until a mix begins to form and the shine dulls (Fig. 2-24).
5. Roll a small amount of the excess acrylic into a ball to evaluate the setting time of the acrylic while the vacuform matrix is in the mouth.
6. Place the mixed acrylic in the area being worked on in the vacuform matrix.

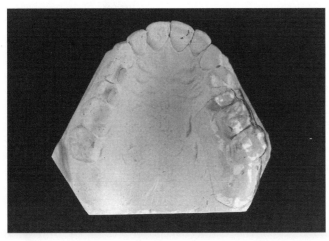

Figure 2-23. Quadrant vacuform matrix shell on a stone model.

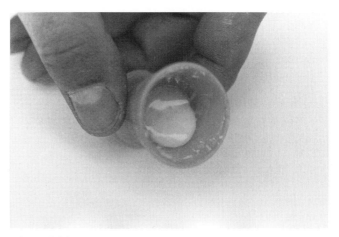

Figure 2-24. Mixed acrylic ready to place in the vacuform matrix.

7. Carefully place the vacuform matrix in the patient's mouth and hold it on the teeth for approximately 1 minute or until the ball of excess acrylic begins to warm (Fig. 2-25).
8. At this point, begin lifting the vacuform matrix off and on the tooth several times.
9. After the acrylic begins to cool, have the patient open and remove the vacuform matrix. The acrylic should have formed to the tooth (Fig. 2-26A,B).
10. Mark the margins with a sharp pencil and avoid this line when trimming.
11. Remove the acrylic from the vacuform matrix, trim the excess acrylic from

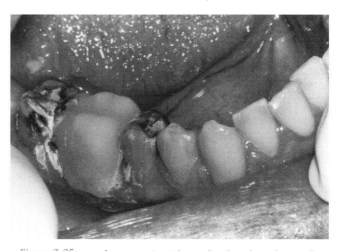

Figure 2-25. Vacuform matrix with acrylic placed on the tooth.

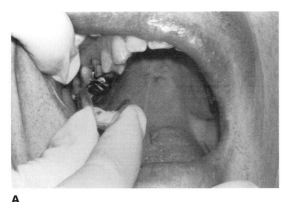 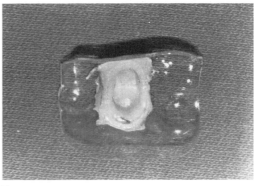

A   **B**

Figure 2-26. (**A,B**) Removing the vacuform matrix from the tooth.

the crown and gingival margins with a slow-speed handpiece and acrylic bur, try temporary crown on the tooth, have the patient bite softly, then remove the acrylic temporary crown.

12. Finish trimming the acrylic temporary crown and polish with wet pumice and rag wheel on the lathe.
13. Check the occlusion with 2×2s and articulating paper on forceps and make adjustments as necessary.
14. Cement the acrylic temporary with temporary cement (Fig. 2-27).
15. Provide postoperative instructions and remove excess cement.
16. Rinse the patient.

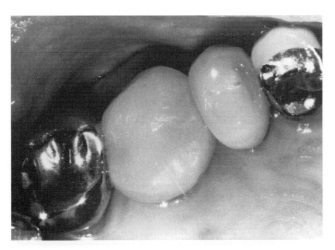

Figure 2-27. Cemented acrylic temporary crown.

Mixing and Delivery of Cements

Another duty of the dental assistant in which consistency is critical is the mixing and delivery of dental cements. Proper mixing gives the doctor adequate working time for placement of the material. Prior to mixing any cement or luting agent, the dental assistant should be familiar with the manufacturer's instructions and recommendations for handling the material. The mixing of the following materials is reviewed:

- zinc phosphate cement and bases
- glass ionomer cements and liners
- IRM sedative filling material
- endodontic sealers

Zinc Phosphate Cement

1. Use 8 drops and a capful of powder (divide in half for single-unit crowns).
2. Divide the powder into four sections, and then divide the first section into four equal sections.
3. Mix the first section of powder with the entire amount of liquid on a cold glass slab (approximately 68°F) over a broad area for 15 seconds.
4. Next, mix in 1/16 section for 15 seconds, then another 1/16 section for 15 seconds, each time incorporating the powder with all of the liquid.
5. Begin mixing the remaining 1/4 sections slowly until you can lift a string of cement off the glass slab with the side of the spatula (Fig. 2-28). Working time is approximately 2 minutes.

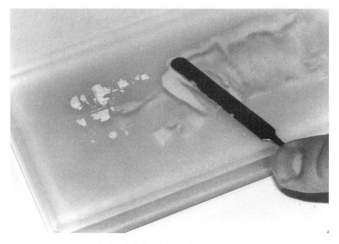

Figure 2-28. Mixing zinc phosphate cement.

6. Fill the crown with cement by lining the internal walls, being careful not to overfill.
7. Place the crown, upside down, on your hand and pass it to the doctor for final placement on the tooth. After several minutes, the cement will harden and is easily removed from the margins with an explorer.

Zinc Phosphate Base

1. The base is mixed the same way as the cement, but more powder is used and mixing continues until the material becomes very stringy.
2. It is then rolled into a ball using additional powder on the dental assistant's gloved fingers.
3. The material is then passed to the doctor on a Woodson plugger or condenser.
4. After the material has been condensed and set, it is cut back to the desired height and depth with hand or high-speed instruments.

Glass Ionomer Cement and Liner

Glass ionomers are available in both light-cure and auto-cure varieties. Unlike zinc phosphate, glass ionomers are mixed thoroughly, without increments, in a 1:1 powder:liquid ratio. Working time is approximately 2 minutes.

1. When mixing, apply on a paper pad with a smooth surface, and incorporate the entire amount of liquid and powder at the same time. If desired, additional powder may be added to develop a thicker mix.
2. The material is then delivered to the doctor on either a pad or a spatula.
3. The doctor uses a plastic or similar placing instrument.
4. The material is then light-cured for approximately 40 seconds if the light-cured variety is used.

IRM Sedative Filling Material

This material is mixed quickly and requires the most force while mixing. Like the zinc phosphate base material, it is rolled into a ball by incorporating a lot of powder (normally 2 drops per 2 scoops of powder).

1. The material should be mixed until the ball no longer sticks to the gloves, then passed to the doctor on a Woodson plugger or condenser.
2. It is then placed in the tooth, condensed, and left to harden.

Endodontic Sealer

This material is mixed quickly with 1 drop of liquid per 1 capsule or scoop of powder on a glass slab.

1. It is mixed to a slightly thinner consistency than zinc phosphate cement.
2. The sealer is placed on the gutta percha filling material and passed to the doctor for placement.

Measuring Endodontic Instruments

Endodontic materials, instruments, and procedures are changing more rapidly than any other area in dentistry. Due to the addition of ultrasonic devices, rotary instruments, greater taper files, and crown-down techniques, the dental assistant has many more challenges staying current with techniques and training.

After the patient has been anesthetized and the tooth isolated with a dental dam, the doctor begins the root canal procedure, including the following steps:

1. The doctor gains access to the pulp chamber.
2. After locating the canal(s) with an endodontic explorer, the doctor extirpates the pulp with a barbed broach.
3. At this time, the dental assistant estimates the working length of the canal from the initial radiograph.
4. The doctor then negotiates the canals with a K-type file, preferably #08 or #10, with a lubricant and an emulsifier such as RC Prep.
5. Once the doctor has found the working length, the dental assistant takes the working length radiograph.
6. When the working length has been confirmed, the dental assistant measures and sets the stoppers on the remaining files.
7. Depending on the cleaning and shaping technique the doctor uses, the dental assistant will set the stoppers on the #10 through #25K files and then step back the #30 through #80 files in succession from the working length.
8. It is important for the dental assistant to irrigate the canals with copious amounts of sodium hypochlorite while the doctor is enlarging the canals.
9. Many doctors prefer to enlarge the canals with a combination of Gates-Glidden drills or even rotary-driven nickel-titanium files.
10. When measuring the various instruments, it is important to continue verifying the lengths and keeping the canals irrigated with sodium hypochlorite.
11. After the doctor has obtained the final shape of the canals, the dental assistant flushes the canals with the irrigating solution and dries them with paper points in preparation for obturation.

Upon completion of the new patient examination, it is necessary for the doctor and the dental assistant to compile the data and formulate the treatment plan. If the initial examination does not give the doctor adequate time or enough information to complete the treatment plan, the patient will need a separate appointment for study models, facebow transfer, and a centric record for occlusal analysis. In general, the proper sequence of treatment will be decided by the doctor, while the appropriate times for the upcoming appointments will be determined by both the doctor and the dental assistant. This information is then given to the financial coordinator, who will discuss the financial arrangements with the patient. The patient then goes to the scheduling coordinator to make the next appointment. Depending on the size of the office, the financial arrangements and scheduling may be handled by the same person or different persons.

In many offices, time is broken up into units. For example, 10 minutes can be equivalent to one unit and six units equal 1 hour. This system was designed for scheduling doctor and assistant time, especially with multiple operatories. The doctor can be in only one place at a time, and with the addition of computerized scheduling, unit scheduling can make the most of everyone's time.

Table 2-1 presents an example of time units for various procedures based on one unit equaling 10 minutes. Table 2-2 presents examples of procedures for a three-operatory office.

TABLE 2-1   Time Units for Various Procedures

Procedure	Appointment Time	Doctor Time
Initial exam	6–9 units	2–3 units
Emergency exam	3–6 units	1–3 units
Amalgam	6 units per quad	3–4 units per quad
Composite	9 units per quad	6–7 units per quad
Crowns	6–9 units	3–5 units
Bridges	12–15 units	9–12 units
Root canals	1 canal—6 units	4–5 units
	2 canals—9 units	6–7 units
	3 or more canals—12 units	8–9 units
Oral surgery	3–4 units per tooth	2–3 units per tooth
Partial and complete dentures	Final impression, 4–6 units	2–3 units
	Max/man relations, 6–9 units	5–7 units
	Clinical try-in, 6–9 units	4–6 units
	Delivery, 4–6 units	2–3 units
Infection control	1 unit per appointment	0 units

TABLE 2-2   Examples of Procedures for a Three-Operatory Office

OP 1 Productive Column	OP 2 Nonproductive Column	OP 3 Hygiene Column
Quadrant dentistry	All exams	Adult recall exam
Amalgams	Crown seats	Scale and prophylaxis
Composites	Small filling	
Crown and bridge	Adjust and polish amalgams	
Root canals	Denture adjustments	
Oral surgery	Child recall exam	

Many textbooks and continuing dental education courses focus on ergonomics, the most efficient operating positions for the dental assistant, doctor, and patient. The following information can be adapted for specific situations but is intended to serve as a general guideline for all dental procedures.

Chair Position

To be comfortable and efficient, the doctor and the dental assistant should sit in an upright position, with the stool adjusted so that the operator's knees are slightly higher than the thighs. Feet should be flat on the floor except for those of the dental assistant, who will most likely rest the feet on the bar of the stool. Many dental chairs have good lumbar support and height and can be adjusted. The dental assistant should sit 4 to 6 inches higher than the doctor in order to see over the doctor's hands. Many dental assistants use the abdominal bar; however, it may lead to many back problems due to poor lumbar support and poor posture.

Operating Zones

There are three zones or working areas in the operatory. The patient is seated in the middle of the room, referred to as zone 1. The doctor, if right-handed, is seated to the right of the patient, usually between the 9 and 12 o'clock positions, in zone 2. The dental assistant is seated to the left of the patient in zone 3 between 1 and 3 o'clock. If the doctor is left-handed, the dental assistant works from the right side, but in our example we will assume that the doctor is right-handed.

Maxillary Arch

When work is being done on the maxillary arch, the patient should be in a supine position. The doctor will usually be seated at 11 to 12 o'clock, working indirectly with a mouth mirror. The dental assistant should be between 2 and 3 o'clock, sitting parallel to the patient but in the opposite direction. When the doctor is using indirect vision, the dental assistant must keep the mouth mirror clean and dry, the operating light extended out and over the patient, and the operating field evacuated.

Mandibular Arch

When working on the mandibular arch, the doctor and the dental assistant attempt to operate using direct vision. The patient is placed all the way down to the floor with the back slightly elevated. This position enables the doctor to operate between the 9 and 12 o'clock positions. The dental assistant should sit toward the 12 o'clock position, with the left knee aligned with the patient's left shoulder, but as the doctor moves toward 9 o'clock, the dental assistant should rotate the knees to face the dentist. This position enables the dental assistant to retract with the air-water tip and still maintain good posture. The operating light for the mandibular arch should be extended over the patient's head, an arm's length away for adequate focal distance, and directed toward the occlusal surface.

Study Questions

1. Topical anesthetic for an inferior alveolar nerve block is placed be-tween the _____ and the _____ approximately _____ cm above the occlusal plane.

2. Topical anesthetic should be held in place for _____ minutes.

3. Dental dam septa can be inverted using _____ and a _____.

4. A dental dam prepared for an endodontic procedure should have how many holes?

5. When placing the HVE, the tip should be _____ to the buccal or lingual surface of the tooth.

6. The _____ grasp is the preferred hand position for the HVE because more _____ is gained.

7. When passing instruments during a procedure, the dental assistant receives the used instrument with which finger?

8. After receiving the used instrument, the dental assistant passes the new instru-ment with the nib _____ when working on maxillary teeth and with the _____ when working on mandibular teeth.

9. When radiographs are taken, the white side of the film packet should be facing the x-ray tube. T or F?

10. When bitewing or periapical radiographs are taken, the film should be placed (buccal or lingual) to the teeth.

11. When the Tofflemire matrix and retainer are placed, the retainer must always rest against the _____ surfaces of the teeth.

12. The opening of the slot on the Tofflemire retainer must always point toward the _____ to facilitate removal.

13. When the daysheet is prepared, each tooth to be restored has its own line with what three pieces of information?

Patient Records/ Chart Entries

Objectives

This chapter presents the basic charts and entries required for treatment documentation. The following chart forms and topics will be covered:

General Information Form

Patient Need Survey/Interview Form

Medical History Form

Dental History Form

Periodontal Form

Initial Clinical Examination Form

Treatment Plan Form

Record of Treatment Form

Laboratory Prescription Forms

Antibiotics and Analgesics

Universal Treatment and Emergency Medications

Consent Form

Referral Forms

This form contains all of the patient's pertinent financial information. The dental assistant should check to be sure that the patient has completed and signed this form for the front office staff. The billing and insurance information will help the financial coordinator to determine the patient's insurance benefits and credit status. Another important question concerns who referred the patient. This is important for marketing purposes but may also provide information on the nature of the new patient.

In this example the patient, Dan Smith, was referred to the office by his brother, Greg. Mr. Smith works for Alaska Airlines and has insurance benefits from Aetna Insurance Company (Fig. 3-1).

GENERAL INFORMATION

REFERED BY: Greg Smith (brother)　　　DATE: 1-3-98

NAME: Dan Smith

RESIDENCE: 1000 Park Avenue　　　CITY: Seattle　　　STATE: WA　　ZIP: 98449

HOME PHONE: 206-632-1000　　BIRTHDATE: 12-10-56　　SOCIAL SECURITY NUMBER: 532-00-0000

OCCUPATION: Flight Attendant　　EMPLOYER: Alaska Airlines

ADDRESS OF EMPLOYER: 1220 Marginal Way　　　　　　WORK PHONE: 206-635-1000

MARRIED:__ SINGLE:__ DIVORCED: X

NAME OF SPOUSE:_____　　SOCIAL SECURITY NUMBER:_____

OCCUPATION:_____　　EMPLOYER:_____

ADDRESS OF EMPLOYER:_____　　WORK PHONE:_____

EMERGENCY PERSON WE CAN CONTACT: Mrs. Smith WORK PHONE: 206-841-5300　HOME PHONE: 840-3200

INSURANCE INFORMATION

	PRIMARY INSURANCE COMPANY	SECONDARY INSURANCE COMPANY
1. Employee's Name	1. Dan Smith	1.
2. Employee's Social Security #	2. 532-00-0000	2.
3. Employee's Sex	3. M	3.
4. Employee's Date of Birth	4. 12-10-56	4.
5. Insurance Co. Name	5. Aetna	5.
6. Insurance Co. Address	6. 1000 Olive Way　City: Seattle	6.　City:
7. Group Plan #	7. 1007A6	7.
8. Local Union #	8. 312	8.
9. Policy #	9. AE56302	9.
10. Employer's Name	10. Alaska Airlines	10.
11. Employer's Address	11. 1220 Marginal Way　City: Seattle	11.　City:
12. Family Members Covered	12.　　NAME　　　BIRTHDATE	12.　　NAME　　　BIRTHDATE

ASSIGNMENT AND RELEASE

I hereby authorize my insurance benefits to be paid directly to the dentist. I am financially responsible for any balances due. I also authorize the dentist to release any information required for this claim. I authorize that my records can be used by the doctor if he so determines.

In consideration of the service rendered to me by this dental office, I am obligated to pay said office in accordance with its credit terms and policy.

I consent to the taking of photographs and x-rays before, during, and after treatment, and to the use of same by the doctor in scientific papers or demonstrations.

I certify that I have read or had read to me the contents of this form and do realize the risks and limitations involved.

SIGNATURE Dan Smith　　　　　DATE 1-3-98

Figure 3-1. General information form.

The patient need survey is an optional form that can be used during the new patient interview. It is not to be filled out by the patient, but rather to be used by the dental assistant to get more information from the patient. The dental assistant does not have to go through the entire list; only pertinent questions should be asked. In general, the main reason for the survey is to determine the patient's chief concern. After all of the data are collected, the dental assistant can report on the patient's concerns, as well as clinical findings, prior to the doctor's examination.

In this example, Mr. Smith's chief concern is that one of his front teeth hurts. Also noted are: 3 years since the last dental visit, minimal dental care in the past, bad dental experience as a child, continuing fear of dental work, and a desire for more lower teeth (Fig. 3-2).

PATIENT NEED SURVEY

NAME Dan Smith   **DATE** 1-3-98

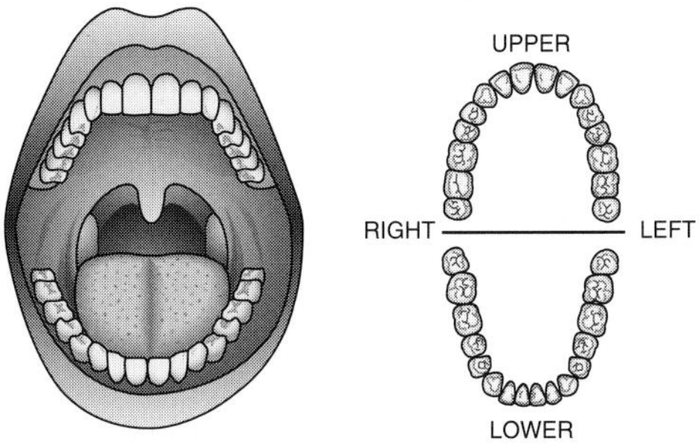

UPPER

RIGHT ———————— LEFT

LOWER

NOTES:

1. Is there anything in particular that you'd like us to take a look at today?
   Pt's front tooth hurts (#8)

2. How long has it been since your last visit?
   3 years

3. What type of dental care have you had in the past?
   Minimal

4. Were those visits relatively comfortable for you?
   Pt. had bad experience as a child – still has fears

5. How do you feel about the results you achieved?

6. How have you been taking care of your mouth at home?

7. How do you feel about your mouth/smile?

8. In addition to the information you have given us, are there any other areas you'd like us to look at today?
   Pt. wants more teeth on the lower Arch

Figure 3-2. Patient need survey.

It is very important to take a thorough medical history from both children and adults. Not only is it safer for the dentist and staff, but there are many medical conditions that the dental team needs to be aware of in treating the patient. Every time the patient comes into the office, his or her medical history should be reviewed, and noted with a date and signature. Patients with heart murmurs, artificial valves, or prostheses should be premedicated with the most current antibiotic regimen according to the American Heart Association. The dental staff should be aware of patients with prior medical conditions such as hypertension, asthma, diabetes, epilepsy, and angina pectoris.

In this example, Mr. Smith is allergic to penicillin and has a heart murmur, diabetes, and epilepsy. Further follow-up will be done with the physician to determine the nature of the heart murmur and the need for antibiotic prophylaxis prior to invasive procedures. Questioning reveals that Mr. Smith's diabetes appears to be adult onset and is diet controlled. He is on no current medication for epilepsy and has not had a petit mal seizure in over 5 years. As a precautionary measure when treating Mr. Smith, the office should have on hand a source of sugar such as canned orange juice or a candy bar. Should a seizure occur, the patient should be placed in a supine position, all objects removed from the mouth, care taken to prevent injury, vital signs monitored, and medical assistance called for if necessary (Fig. 3-3).

MEDICAL HISTORY

Patient Name___Dan Smith_____
Date of Birth___12-10-56_____   Last Complete Medical Exam___9-30-96_____

Family Physician___Dr. Jones_____	Speciality _General_____
Address___3200 Meridian Street, Puyallup WA_____	Phone_845-2100_____
Additional Physician_____	Speciality_____
Address_____	Phone_____

1. Have you taken any medications in the last two years?___No_____
2. List all medications you are currently taking___N/A_____

3. Are you aware of having an allergic (**or adverse reaction**) to any medication or
   substance? If yes, please list___Penicillin_____
4. Have you been hospitalized during the past five years?__No_____
5. Please **circle** all of the following conditions you have had, or have at present.

Heart (Surgery, Disease, Attack)	Supervised Diet	Hepatitis A, B, other
Chest Pain/Angina Pectoris	(Diabetes)	Liver Disease/Jaundice
Congenital Heart Disease	Ulcers	HIV Positive/AIDS
(Heart Murmur)	Glaucoma	Communicable Disease
High Blood Pressure	Thyroid Disease	Kidney Trouble
Mitral Valve Prolapse	Emphysema	Anemia
Artificial Heart Valve	Chronic Cough	Blood Disorder
Heart Pacemaker	Tuberculosis	Drug Dependency
Shortness of Breath	Asthma	Alcohol Dependency
Rheumatic Fever	Hay Fever	Tobacco Dependency
Scarlet Fever	Latex Sensitivity	Nervous/Anxious
Arthritis/Rheumatism	Allergies or Hives	Neurological Disorders
Cortisone Medicine	Sinus Trouble	(Epilepsy) or Seizures
Swollen Ankles	Cancer/Tumors	Fainting or Dizzy Spells
Stroke	Radiation/Chemotherapy	Psychiatric/Psychological Care
Artificial Joints (Hip, Knee, etc.)		

6. Do you use more than two pillows to sleep?__No_____
7. Have you lost or gained more than 10 pounds in the past year?__No_____
8. Do you have, or have you had any disease, condition, or problem not listed? If yes,
   please list__No_____
WOMEN: Are you: **Pregnant?** Yes,___Months No   **Nursing?** Yes No
                        Taking Birth Control Pills? Yes No

I understand that the above information is necessary to provide me with dental care in a safe and efficient manner. I have answered all questions to the best of my knowledge. Should further information be needed, you have my permission to ask the respective health care provider or agency, who may release such information to you. I will notify the doctor of any change in my health or medication.

Patient/Guardian Signature___Dan Smith_____   Date__1-3-98_____

History Review
Pt. allergic to penicillin
Check status of heart murmur w/physician, premedicate
w/E-mycin prior to perio probings, cleanings, etc.
Diabetes is adult onset and diet controlled
No current meds. for epilepsy, last petit mal seizure 5+ years

Dates Reviewed___1-3-98____   _GMS_____

Figure 3-3. Medical history form.

Previous dental experiences are important to know about so that a concerted effort can be made to avoid a bad experience. The dental history form should also include questions about temporomandibular joint (TMJ) disorders or other oral habits such as bruxism. After the questions are reviewed, it should be easier to determine the patient's dental IQ and educate the patient accordingly. The dental history will also let the dental staff know if the patient has had any teeth extracted or if the patient has seen an orthodontist or another specialist. The chief concern of the patient will also be noted on this form.

In this example, the patient's immediate dental concern is that his front tooth hurts. Also noted is the bad experience he had as a child in having a tooth removed without anesthesia, concerns about periodontal disease, missing teeth and unhappiness with the appearance of the teeth, and interest in retaining the remainder of his teeth. Further follow-up on "jaw popping" or TMJ noise may also be necessary. These and other significant findings during the patient interview can be summarized in the "Notes" section (Fig. 3-4).

DENTAL HISTORY

Previous Dentisit_____ Period of Treatment_____ Specialty_____
Address_____ Phone_____

Last dental visit_____ Last full-mouth x-ray_____ Last complete dental exam_____
What is your immediate dental concern? _front tooth hurts_____

Please encircle **YES** or **NO**. If YES, please fill in details.

(Yes) No   Are you presently in any dental pain? _Front tooth_____
Yes (No)   Is any part of your mouth sensitive to temperature, pressure, food or drink?_____
(Yes) No   Have you ever experienced any unfavorable reaction to dentistry?_____
              What? _As a child I had a tooth removed without being numb_____
Yes (No)   Have you ever had a bad reaction to a dental anesthetic? When?_____

Yes (No)   Do you have any growths or swellings in your mouth? How long have they existed?_____
Yes (No)   Do you have any difficulty in swallowing?_____
Yes (No)   Do you have a burning sensation of your mouth?_____

(Yes) No   Do your gums bleed when brushing your mouth?_____
Yes (No)   Do you avoid brushing any part of your mouth?_____
Yes (No)   Have you ever been told you have pyorrhea? When?_____
(Yes) No   Does food catch between your teeth? _I lost a tooth on my upper left_____
(Yes) No   Do you have an unpleasant taste or odor in your mouth?_____

Yes (No)   Do you have any pain or soreness around your eyes or ears or other parts of your face?_____
              What?_____
Yes (No)   Are you aware of stiff neck muscles? How often?_____
Yes (No)   Do you ever awaken with an awareness of your teeth or jaws? How often?_____
Yes (No)   Are you aware of clenching your teeth during your daytime hours? How often?_____
Yes (No)   Have you ever been told you grind your teeth during sleep? How often?_____
(Yes) No   Are you aware of your jaw clicking or (popping) while eating or yawning? How often?_____
Yes (No)   Do you have difficulty in opening your mouth widely?_____
Yes (No)   Do you have "tension" headaches? How often?_____

(Yes) No   Have you lost any teeth? From what cause? _I got in a fight_____
(Yes) No   Do any members of your family including your parents wear dentures?_____
(Yes) No   Do you feel you will eventually wear full artificial dentures?_____

(Yes) No   Are you dissatisfied with with your teeth and their appearance?_____
Yes (No)   Have you ever had orthodontic treatment?_____
Yes (No)   Do you think your dental disease is active?_____
(Yes) No   Do you want to learn to control your dental disease and retain your teeth?_____
(Yes) No   Are you deeply concerned about the finances required to return your mouth to excellent dental
              health?_____

Notes

      C.C.-front tooth hurts
      bad experience as child
      periodontal concerns
      missing teeth and unhappy w/appearance
      wants to retain teeth

Figure 3-4. Dental history form.

Periodontal Form

The periodontal form should be clear and easy to read. It should have many spaces for dated consecutive probings. Many offices use the color red to denote periodontal pocket depths of 4 mm or more and blue to denote pocket depths less than 4 mm. It is a good idea for the dental assistant to prepare the patient for the periodontal probings that the dentist or dental hygienist will be recording. By discussing periodontal disease and the measurements, the dental assistant will decrease the amount of doctor time required for education during the new patient examination.

In this example, the patient had initial periodontal probings on January 3, 1997. In practice, as mentioned above, periodontal pocket depths of 4 mm or more would be recorded in red and pocket depths of less than 4 mm in blue. Missing teeth #1, 13, 16, 17, 18, 30, 31, and 32 have been crossed out on both the tooth chart and the probing spaces (Fig. 3-5).

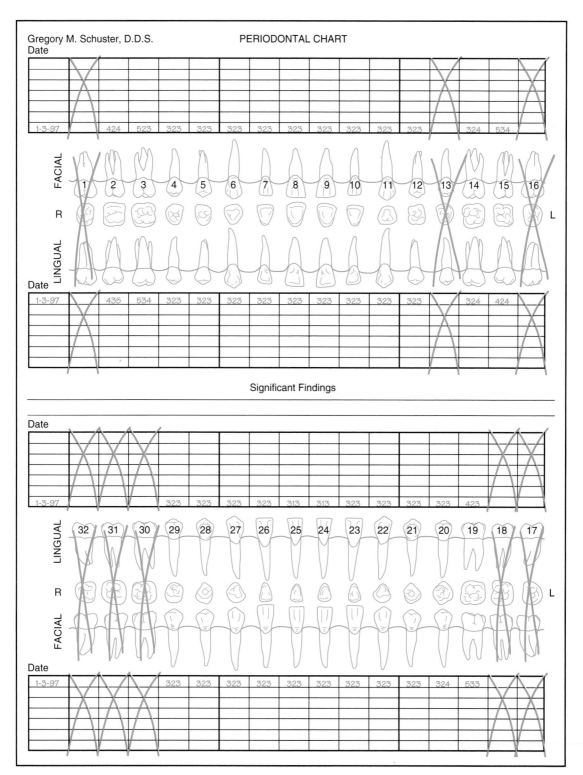

Gregory M. Schuster, D.D.S.   PERIODONTAL CHART

Figure 3-5. Periodontal form.

Initial Clinical Examination Form

The initial clinical examination form should contain a tooth chart that the dental assistant will fill out in blue pencil, recording the existing conditions and restorations of the patient. During the examination, any decay or significant oral findings noted by the doctor are charted in red pencil on the same form. A thorough TMJ form is very important in diagnosing the patient's current status and in providing records when taking study models for occlusal analysis. A head and neck examination, as part of an oral cancer screening examination, should be performed, as well as a periodontal and radiographic examination.

In this example, the patient's vital signs, existing restorations, current restorative needs, and TMJ and occlusal findings have been recorded in the appropriate colors (Fig. 3-6).

INITIAL CLINICAL EXAMINATION

PATIENT NAME Dan Smith	WISHES TO BE CALLED Danny
PATIENT ACCOUNT NO.	DATE 1-3-98

VITAL SIGNS:	Blood Pressure 128/85	Pulse 60

3 unit Bridge

W   O

R | L

A B C D E   F G H I J

T S R Q P   O N M L K

/RPD

DENTAL IQ   I II III IV V

EMOTIONAL MOTIVATORS	EMOTIONAL CONCERNS
☐ ESTHETIC _____	☐ FEAR _____
☐ HEALTH _____	☐ PAIN (CONCERN) _____
☐ PREVENTION _____	☐ MONEY _____
☐ FUNCTION _____	☐ TIME _____
☐ PAIN (MOTIVATOR) _____	☐ EMBARRASSMENT _____
☐ GUILT _____	☐ ANGER _____
☐ STATUS _____	☐ FRUSTRATION _____
☐ PEER PRESSURE _____	☐ OTHER _____
☐ OTHER _____	

COMMENTS _____
_____
_____
_____

INITIAL TMJ

☐ MUSCULATURE _____
☐ PAIN L R _____
☐ CREPITUS L R _____
☒ POPPING (L) (R) _____
☐ MAXIMUM OPENING (UNASSISTED) _____ 48 _____ mm
☐ DEVIATION UPON OPENING _____ L _____ R _____ None

_____
_____
_____

INITIAL OCCLUSION

DENTAL   Class _I_   Division _____
SKELETAL   Class _____
OVERJET _3_ mm   OVERBITE _4_ mm
SLIDE _____ mm   MIDLINE _____
PROFILE _____   CROSSBITE _____
MOLAR RELATION: L _____   R _____
CUSPID RELATION: L _____   R _____
HABITS: Thumb   Tongue   Other _____

_____
_____

Figure 3-6. Initial clinical examination form. Reproduced courtesy of the PRIDE Institute.

SOFT TISSUE EXAM

DATE	WNL									
FACE	WNL									
NECK										
LYMPH NODES										
LIPS										
BUCCAL MUCOSA										
FLOOR OF MOUTH										
TONGUE										
HARD PALATE										
SOFT PALATE										
ORO PHARYNX										
SALIVARY GLANDS										
STAFF INITIALS	√									

INITIAL SOFT TISSUE EXAM

Left   Right   Front

COMMENTS _____

_____
_____
_____
_____
_____
_____
_____
_____
_____
_____

INITIAL PERIODONTAL EXAM (please circle)

		CLINICAL IMPRESSION:	Within Normal Limits
INFLAMMATION:	NONE LIGHT MODERATE SEVERE		
EXUDATE:	NONE BLOOD SUPPURATION		Type 1 Gingivitis Type 3 Moderate
ATTACHED GINGIVA:	PINK RED MAGENTA		Type 2 Incipient Type 4 Advanced
	STIPPLED GLOSSY GRANULAR		Early onset periodontitis: localized generalized
CONSISTENCY:	FIRM BOGGY FIBROUS		Periodontitis assoc. with systemic disease
MARGINS:	THIN SWOLLEN RECEDED IRREGULAR		Acute Necrotizing ulcerative gingivitis
PAPILLAE:	POINTED BLUNTED FLAT INVERTED		Refractory periodontitis

ATTACHED GINGIVA: PINK   RED   MAGENTA

FIRM   BOGGY   FIBROUS

CALCULUS: NONE   LIGHT   MODERATE   HEAVY

SUPRAGINGIVAL   SUBGINGIVAL

ORAL HYGIENE: GOOD   FAIR   POOR

COMMENTS _____
_____
_____
_____
_____

INITIAL RADIOGRAPHY EXAM

BONE LOSS _____ BONY LESIONS _____   COMMENTS _____

FURCATIONS _____ IMPACTIONS _____   _____

UNFAVORABLE C/R RATIO _____   _____

TOOTH DEVELOPMENT _____   _____

OTHER _____   _____

Figure 3-6. Continued

Like the initial clinical examination form, this form should have a tooth chart for recording restorative needs in red pencil. When restorations are completed, they are filled in with blue pencil. When determining the sequence of treatment, the treatment plan form is divided into four categories:

- Emergent care: the patient's pain is relieved through extractions, root canals, and/or incision and drainage. Medical referrals for systemic disease noted during the new patient examination also take place at this time.
- Treatment and stabilization of periodontal disease.
- Restoration of dental caries.
- Definitive treatment including crowns, bridges, implants, dentures, cosmetic work, and referrals to orthodontists and other specialists. Such treatment is performed only when the periodontal condition has stabilized and the patient is caries free.

In this example, the treatment plan has been formulated according to the four categories listed above. The appointments are numbered, with the appropriate time units listed for the scheduling coordinator (Fig. 3-7).

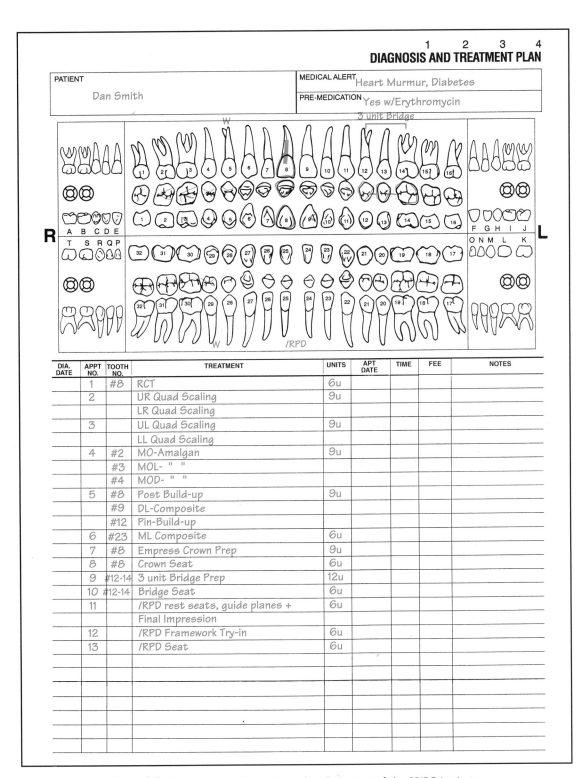

DIAGNOSIS AND TREATMENT PLAN

1   2   3   4

PATIENT
Dan Smith

MEDICAL ALERT Heart Murmur, Diabetes

PRE-MEDICATION Yes w/Erythromycin

3 unit Bridge

R   A B C D E   T S R Q P

L   F G H I J   O N M L K

W   /RPD

DIA. DATE	APPT NO.	TOOTH NO.	TREATMENT	UNITS	APT DATE	TIME	FEE	NOTES
	1	#8	RCT	6u				
	2		UR Quad Scaling	9u				
			LR Quad Scaling					
	3		UL Quad Scaling	9u				
			LL Quad Scaling					
	4	#2	MO-Amalgan	9u				
		#3	MOL- " "					
		#4	MOD- " "					
	5	#8	Post Build-up	9u				
		#9	DL-Composite					
		#12	Pin-Build-up					
	6	#23	ML Composite	6u				
	7	#8	Empress Crown Prep	9u				
	8	#8	Crown Seat	6u				
	9	#12-14	3 unit Bridge Prep	12u				
	10	#12-14	Bridge Seat	6u				
	11		/RPD rest seats, guide planes +	6u				
			Final Impression					
	12		/RPD Framework Try-in	6u				
	13		/RPD Seat	6u				

Figure 3-7. Treatment plan form. Reproduced courtesy of the PRIDE Institute.

Record of Treatment Form

For every chart entry, the dental assistant should record the following information:

- date
- tooth numbers
- tooth surfaces
- anesthetic used (type and amount)
- restorative material used
- procedure done (liners, pins, posts)
- prescriptions given
- any instructions the doctor has given to the patient regarding informed consent or any complications

The dental assistant should also note any important conversation between the patient and doctor, and record the next appointment. The form should have the dental assistant's signature or initials. Figures 3-8 to 3-23 show typical write-ups for various procedures recorded on the record of treatment form.

PATIENT NAME			**RECORD OF TREATMENT**		
PATIENT ACCOUNT NO.					
DATE	TOOTH	SURFACE	PROCEDURE	INIT.	FEE
1/3/98			Patient (Pt.) presented to office for new patient exam with (w/)		
			chief concern of front tooth hurting. Review health history (hx),		
			recorded vital signs on Initial Clinical Examination form, and took		
			full mouth series (FMX) of radiographs. Doctor (Dr.) discussed		
			need for root canal treatment (RCT) on tooth #8 to be started		
			as soon as possible.		
			N.A.: #8 RCT-Open and medicate	G.J.W.	

Figure 3-8. New patient examination procedure.

DATE	TOOTH	SURFACE	PROCEDURE	INIT.	FEE
			RECORD OF TREATMENT		
			PATIENT NAME		
			PATIENT ACCOUNT NO.		
1/3/98			Pt. presents w/pain & swelling upper anterior (UA) area. Took		
			periapical radiograph (PAX) tooth #7. Tooth #7 was cold and		
			percussion sensitive (sens.) and exhibited a periapical lesion on		
			the radiograph. The lesion was determined to be of endodontic		
			origin (LEO) and the Dr. gave options for RCT or extraction (TE)		
			#7. Pt. opted for RCT. Gave 1 carpule (carp.) 2% lidocaine		
			w/1:100,000 epinephrine anesthetic (2% lido/1:100,000 epi),		
			open & broach #7 and established working length (WL)		
			WL: 21mm to #25K file		
			Irrigated w/sodium hypochlorite, dried w/paper points, placed		
			CMCP cotton pellet (cp), and CAVIT temporary (temp.).		
			Rx: Vicodin; 6 tabs, 1 tab q3-4h prn pain, no refill		
			Rx: Keflex 500 mg; 29 tabs, 2 tabs stat then 1 tab q6h until		
			gone, no refill Dr. informed pt. to go to emergency room if		
			swelling increases and to call if any problems occur.		
			N.A.: #7 RCT-Instrument & fill	G.J.W.	

Figure 3-9. Emergency examination and root canal open and medicate procedure.

RECORD OF TREATMENT

PATIENT NAME

PATIENT ACCOUNT NO.

DATE	TOOTH	SURFACE	PROCEDURE	INIT.	FEE
1/5/98			Pt. presents for fillings on upper left (UL) but wanted ones on		
			lower right (LR) done first due to cold sens. Gave 2 carps		
			2% lido/1:100,000 epi inferior alveolar and long buccal (IA & LB)		
	#29	MOD-A			
	#30	MOD-A	deep caries, Vitrebond liner placed		
	#31	MO-A			
			Dr. informed pt. of deep decay #30 and possibility (poss.) of		
			RCT in the future. Also explained poss. of long term cold sens.		
			but to call if severe pain or swelling develops.		
			N.A.: #9 DL-C, #10 MF-C, #11 ML-C	G.M.S.	

Figure 3-10. Amalgam procedure.

RECORD OF TREATMENT

PATIENT NAME

PATIENT ACCOUNT NO.

DATE	TOOTH	SURFACE	PROCEDURE	INIT.	FEE
1/6/98			Pt. presents for anterior composites. Gave 3 carps 2%		
			lido/1:100,000 epi, etch w/37% phosphoric acid, prime and bond		
			w/One-Step, fill w/Z-100 shade A3.		
	#9	DL-C			
	#10	MF-C			
	#11	ML-C			
			N.A.: #19 PFC Prep, Imp., Temp.	G.J.W.	

Figure 3-11. Composite procedure.

DATE	TOOTH	SURFACE	PROCEDURE	INIT.	FEE
			PATIENT NAME		
			PATIENT ACCOUNT NO.		
			RECORD OF TREATMENT		
1/7/98			Pt. presents for crown #19. Took PAX #19 of post build-up. Gave		
			2 carps 2% lido/1:100,000 epi (IA & LB) check occlusion, alginate		
			impression (imp.) taken for temp., shade A3.5 gingival/A2 incisal.		
			Prep, imp., bite registration (reg.), acrylic temp. cemented (cem.)		
			w/Temp-Bond. Dr. informed pt. of poss. sens. around gumline.		
	#19		PFC Prep, Imp., Temp.		
			N.A.: #19 PFC Seat	G.M.S.	

Figure 3-12. Crown and bridge preparation procedure.

DATE	TOOTH	SURFACE	PROCEDURE	INIT.	FEE
			PATIENT NAME		
			PATIENT ACCOUNT NO.		
			RECORD OF TREATMENT		
1/25/98			Pt. presents for delivery of crown #19. No anesthetic given, temp.		
			removed, tooth cleaned w/cp, Dr. checked contacts, margins, and		
			adjusted occlusion (adj. occl.), polish & cem. w/Vitremer luting		
			cement.		
	#19	PFC	Seat		
			Dr. informed pt. of poss. cold sens. and to call if bite feels high.		
			Pt. was happy w/shade & fit.		
			N.A.: #30 PFC Prep, Imp., Temp.	G.M.S.	

Figure 3-13. Crown and bridge seat procedure.

RECORD OF TREATMENT

PATIENT NAME					
PATIENT ACCOUNT NO.					

DATE	TOOTH	SURFACE	PROCEDURE	INIT.	FEE
1/7/98			Pt. presents for finish of RCT #7. Gave 1 carp 2% lido/1:100,000		
			epi. Removed temp., verified WL at 21mm & instrumented to		
			#60K file, irrigated w/sodium hypochlorite, dried w/paper points,		
			and filled to WL w/gutta percha (g.p.). Removed all but last 4mm		
			of g.p. w/0.036" and 0.040" Parapost drills and cem. 0.040"		
			post w/Fleck's. Placed composite build-up and informed pt. that		
			crown should be done in the near future.		
	#7	RCT	1 Canal		
	#7	B.U.-C			
			N.A.: #7 PFC Prep, Imp., Temp.	G.J.W.	

Figure 3-14. Root canal obturation and post buildup procedure.

RECORD OF TREATMENT

PATIENT NAME					
PATIENT ACCOUNT NO.					

DATE	TOOTH	SURFACE	PROCEDURE	INIT.	FEE
1/8/98			Pt. presents for final impression for lower partial denture. Dr.		
			prepared guide planes and rest seats and took final imp.		
			w/alginate. Took opposing imp. w/alginate, bite reg., shade A2,		
			mould T-56.		
			/RPD Final Imp.		
			N.A.: /RPD Framework Try-in	G.M.S.	

Figure 3-15. Removable partial denture final impressions procedure.

DATE	TOOTH	SURFACE	PROCEDURE	INIT.	FEE
			PATIENT NAME		
			PATIENT ACCOUNT NO.		
1/22/98			Pt. presents for lower partial denture framework try-in. Dr.		
			evaluated fit and took another bite reg. Ready for teeth set-up		
			and processing.		
			/RPD Framework Try-In		
			N.A.: /RPD Delivery	G.M.S.	

RECORD OF TREATMENT

Figure 3-16. Removable partial denture framework try-in procedure.

DATE	TOOTH	SURFACE	PROCEDURE	INIT.	FEE
			PATIENT NAME		
			PATIENT ACCOUNT NO.		
1/27/98			Pt. presents for delivery of lower partial denture. Dr. evaluated		
			fit and adj. occl. of /RPD. Dr. informed pt. that sore spots may		
			develop and to remove partial denture while sleeping.		
			/RPD Delivery		
			N.A.: 3-day post-op adjustment	G.M.S.	

RECORD OF TREATMENT

Figure 3-17. Removable partial denture delivery procedure.

DATE	TOOTH	SURFACE	PROCEDURE	INIT.	FEE
			RECORD OF TREATMENT		
			PATIENT NAME		
			PATIENT ACCOUNT NO.		
1/4/98			Pt. presents for final impression for upper denture. Dr. took		
			maxillary final impression w/Impregum in custom acrylic tray,		
			facebrow transfer, and bite reg. Took opposing imp. w/alginate,		
			shade A3, mould T-65.		
			CD/ Final Imp.		
			N.A.: CD/ Maxillary/Mandibular Relations	G.J.W.	

Figure 3-18. Complete denture final impression procedure.

DATE	TOOTH	SURFACE	PROCEDURE	INIT.	FEE
			RECORD OF TREATMENT		
			PATIENT NAME		
			PATIENT ACCOUNT NO.		
1/11/98			Pt. presents for maxillary/mandibular relations appointment. Dr.		
			tried in maxillary occlusion rim, checked Camper's plane, vertical		
			dimension at rest (VDR), vertical dimensions of occlusion (VDO),		
			tooth-lip relationship, overjet, midline, and took another bite reg.		
			N.A.: CD/ Clinical Try-in	G.M.S.	

Figure 3-19. Complete denture maxillary/mandibular relations procedure.

			RECORD OF TREATMENT		
PATIENT NAME					
PATIENT ACCOUNT NO.					
DATE	TOOTH	SURFACE	PROCEDURE	INIT.	FEE
1/15/98			Pt. presents for CD/clinical try-in with set-up in wax. Dr. tried in		
			maxillary occlusion rim, checked Camper's plane, VDR, VDO,		
			tooth-lip relationship, overjet, and midline. Pt. pleased with		
			esthetics and ready for delivery.		
			X _____		
			N.A.: CD/ Delivery	G.M.S.	

Figure 3-20. Complete denture clinical try-in procedure.

			RECORD OF TREATMENT		
PATIENT NAME					
PATIENT ACCOUNT NO.					
DATE	TOOTH	SURFACE	PROCEDURE	INIT.	FEE
1/18/98			Pt. presents for delivery of upper denture. Dr. evaluated fit,		
			checked internal of denture for rough spots w/PIP paste,		
			and adj. occl. Dr. informed pt. that sore spots may develop and		
			to remove denture while sleeping.		
			CD/ Delivery		
			N.A.: 3-day post-op adjustment	G.M.S.	

Figure 3-21. Complete denture delivery procedure.

PATIENT NAME					
PATIENT ACCOUNT NO.			**RECORD OF TREATMENT**		
DATE	TOOTH	SURFACE	PROCEDURE	INIT.	FEE
1/8/98			Pt. presents for removal of tooth #16. Reviewed health hx., took		
			vital signs: BP 120/80, Pulse 65, Respirations 16. Gave 2 carps		
			2% lido/1:100,000 epi. Elevated tooth w/Potts elevator and		
			delivered w/212 forceps. Explained post-op instructions and gave		
			pt. written copy.		
			Rx: Vicodin 6 tabs; 1 tab q3-4h prn pain		
	#16	TE			
			N.A.: 6 month recall	G.M.S.	

Figure 3-22. Oral surgery procedure.

PATIENT NAME					
PATIENT ACCOUNT NO.			**RECORD OF TREATMENT**		
DATE	TOOTH	SURFACE	PROCEDURE	INIT.	FEE
1/9/98			Pt. presents for 6 month check-up visit.		
			Exam, 4 BW's, prophy & fluoride		
			Light plaque w/LA supra, subgingival calculus. Oral hygiene		
			instruction (OHI) reviewed, pocket depths recorded and stable.		
			Gave patient new toothbrush (tb) and floss.		
			N.A.: 6 month recall	G.J.W.	

Figure 3-23. Recall appointment.

Laboratory prescription forms are used to record communication between the doctor and the laboratory technician. They can be used for both fixed and removable prosthodontic procedures. In the first example, the doctor has prepared tooth #19 for a porcelain crown fused to metal. The shade, type of metal, porcelain coverage, collar type, occlusal pattern, and specific characterization have been requested (Fig. 3-24). In the second example, the patient is to receive a full upper denture. The shade and mould for the teeth have been requested (Fig. 3-25).

TWIN LAKES DENTAL LABORATORY, INC.
Work Authorization Form

Inv. # _____

Date _____1-7-98_____   Due Date _____

PATIENT ___Dan Smith___   DENTIST ___SCHUSTER___

Age ___38___ Sex: (M) F   License # ___9999___

BONE STRUCTURE: Deli Med (Vigor)   Signature _____

Please fabricate
PFC #19
shade A3.5 gingival 1/3
A2 incisal 2/3

Thanks!

MATERIALS TO BE USED:

_____ T-2 Low Fusion Gold
_____ T-3 Low Fusion Gold
_____ 85% Precious
___✓___ 51% Semi-Precious
_____ InCeram
_____ Porcelain Inlay or Veneers
_____ Dentacolor
___✓___ Full porcelain coverage
_____ Full metal coverage
_____ ½ occ. metal coverage
_____ Metal collar
___✓___ Metal & porcelain collar
_____ Porcelain shoulder
_____ Splinted

OCCLUSION:

_____ Working
___✓___ Incisal guidance
_____ Protrusive
_____ Lateral Protrusive
_____ Ant. guide table
_____ Reshape opposing?

SHADE DESCRIPTION & CHARACTERIZATION

BASE SHADE ___A3.5 ging/A2 inc.___

BODY TRANSLUCENCY   INCISAL TRANS.

Deep _____   Deep _____
Mod. ___✓___   Mod. ___✓___
Shallow _____   Shallow _____

MODIFICATIONS

_____ Chroma _____ More _____ Less
_____ Hue _____ More _____ Less
_____ Value _____ Higher _____ Lower

CHARACTERIZATION

_____ Stained checkline
_____ Enamel crack
_____ Hypocalcification
_____ Interprox coloration
_____ Incisal halo
_____ Occlusal coloration
_____ White cusp tip
_____ Worn incisal
_____ Metallic restoration
_____ Anterior restoration
_____ Gingival coloration
___✓___ Root Simulation
_____ Translucent rod
_____ Pink spot
_____ Highlighting line
_____ Random discoloration

SURFACE GLAZE   SURFACE TEXTURE

_____ High   _____ Smooth
___✓___ Moderate   ___✓___ Moderate
_____ Low   _____ Heavy (stippled)

FLUORESCENCE (Pearl Effect)

COMMENTS _____

Figure 3-24. Laboratory prescription form. Reproduced courtesy of Twin Lakes Dental Laboratory, Tacoma, Washington.

Figure 3-25. Laboratory prescription form. Reproduced courtesy of Tillicum Dental Lab. Inc., Tacoma, Washington.

TILLICUM DENTAL LAB, INC.
"THE MEASURE OF QUALITY"

8409 Spruce St. S.W.
Tacoma, WA 98498
588-2721

DUE DATE

PROCEDURE	DATE	HOUR
try-in	1/15	9AM
FINISH		

Patients Name _John Doe_

Shade _A3_

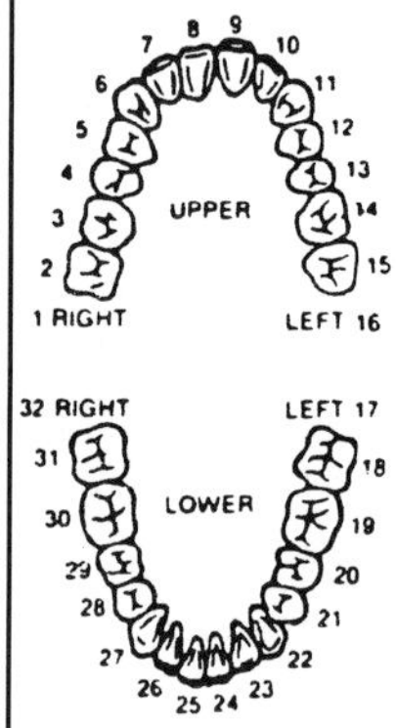

SPECIAL INSTRUCTIONS

Please fabricate

CD/ for clinical

wax try-in.

Mould T-65

Thanks!

SIGNATURE

LICENSE NO
9999

Antibiotics and Analgesics

Common Antibiotics

Antibiotic	Dosage	Schedule
Penicillin VK	500 mg	1q6h
Amoxicillin	500 mg	1q6h
Cephalosporin (Keflex)	500 mg	1q6h
Erythromycin	500 mg	1q6h

Antibiotic Prophylaxis to Prevent Subacute Bacterial Endocarditis

Antibiotic	Dosage	Schedule
Amoxicillin	500 mg	4tabs 1h before dental treatment
Clindamycin	300 mg	2tabs 1h before dental treatment

Substitutes for Penicillin Allergy (Erythromycin, Keflex)

Antibiotic	Dosage	Schedule
Cephalexin	500 mg	4tabs 1h before dental treatment
Azithromycin	250 mg	2tabs 1h before dental treatment

Common Analgesics and Dosages

Mild Pain		
Analgesic	Dosage	Schedule
Aspirin	325 mg	2–3q4h
Ibuprofen (Advil, Motrin, Nuprin)	200 mg	2–4q4h up to 16 tabs/day
Acetaminophen (Tylenol)	325 mg	2–3q4h

Moderate Pain

Analgesic	Dosage	Schedule
Ibuprofen	400–600 mg	1q4h
Tylenol III	(30 mg codeine + 300 mg acetaminophen)	1q4h
Vicodin	(5 mg hydrocodone + 500 mg acetaminophen)	1q4h
Talwin	(25 mg pentazocine + 650 mg aspirin)	1q4h

Severe Pain

Analgesic	Dosage	Schedule
Ibuprofen	800 mg	1q4h
Demerol	50 mg	1q4h
Percodan	(5 mg oxycodone + 325 mg aspirin)	1q4h
Percocet	(5 mg oxycodone + 300 mg acetaminophen)	1q4h
Tylox	(5 mg oxycodone + 500 mg acetaminophen)	1q4h

The following prescriptions are for a broad-spectrum antibiotic (Fig. 3-26) and for moderate pain management (Fig. 3-27).

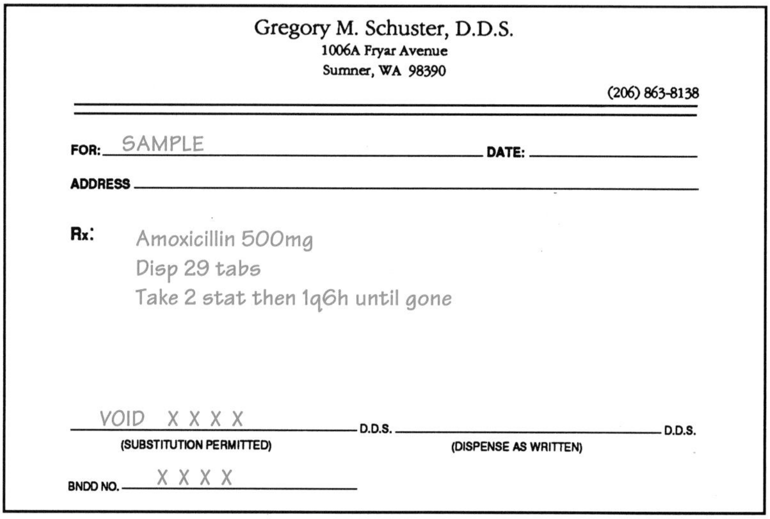

Gregory M. Schuster, D.D.S.
1006A Fryar Avenue
Sumner, WA 98390
(206) 863-8138

FOR: SAMPLE   DATE:

ADDRESS

Rx: Amoxicillin 500mg
     Disp 29 tabs
     Take 2 stat then 1q6h until gone

VOID X X X X _____ D.D.S. _____ D.D.S.
(SUBSTITUTION PERMITTED)   (DISPENSE AS WRITTEN)

BNDD NO. X X X X

Figure 3-26. Prescription for a commonly used broad-spectrum antibiotic.

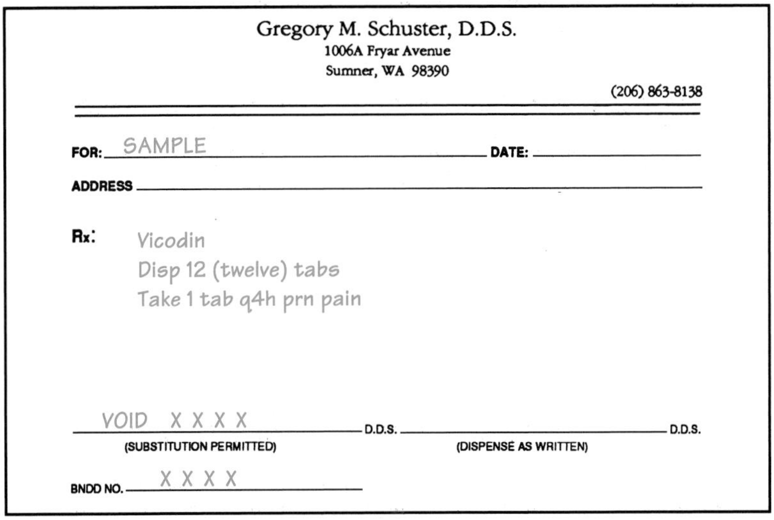

Gregory M. Schuster, D.D.S.
1006A Fryar Avenue
Sumner, WA 98390

(206) 863-8138

FOR: SAMPLE _____ **DATE:** _____

ADDRESS _____

Rx: Vicodin
Disp 12 (twelve) tabs
Take 1 tab q4h prn pain

VOID X X X X
_____ D.D.S. _____ D.D.S.
(SUBSTITUTION PERMITTED)   (DISPENSE AS WRITTEN)

BNDD NO. ___ X X X X _____

Figure 3-27. Prescription for moderate pain management.

Universal Treatment and Emergency Medications

Universal Treatment of Emergencies

1. Place patient in supine position.
2. Open the airway.
3. Monitor vital signs.
4. Call the Emergency Medical Service (911).
5. Provide symptomatic treatment.
6. Transport by EMS.

Medications for Emergencies

Emergency	Medication	Dosage
Cardiac arrest	1:1000 epinephrine IV	0.3–0.5 mg
Anaphylactic reaction	1:1000 epinephrine IV	0.3–1.0 mg
Hypotension	ephedrine	10–50 mg/cc
Bradycardia	atropine	0.4–1.0 mg
Allergies	benadryl	25–50 mg
Angina pectoris	nitroglycerin	0.3-mg tablets
Seizure	diazepam	5 mg/cc
Narcotic overdose	naloxone	0.4 mg/cc

Consent Form

The following is a patient consent form for the following procedures: periodontal condition, root canal procedures, oral surgery procedures, removable prosthodontic procedures, orthodontic procedures, and radiography. Appropriate material should be explained before the patient signs the form (Fig. 3-28).

CONSENT

PERIO _____ This certifies that I, the patient, have been informed of my periodontal (gum) condition. My treatment of choice is:

     ____Referral to a periodontist (gum specialist) at this time.

     ____Maintenance therapy involving regular _____ month cleaning.

         ____With a referral to a periodontist if my condition worsens.

         ____With no referral at any time.

        Signature _____ Date _____

ENDO _#8_ I understand that my tooth is in need of a Root Canal Procedure. I have been informed that complications of pain and infection can occur, and that a small percentage (less than 5%) need retreatment or referral to an Endodontic specialist.

        SignatureX_ _Dan Smith_____ Date _1-17-97_

EXTRACTION _____ I understand that there are occasional risks associated with having teeth extracted which include: movement or drifting of other teeth, drysocket, temporary or permanent numbness, pain or infection. I also understand if sutures are used, I must return to have them removed.

        Signature _____ Date _____

(PARTIAL)/COMPLETE DENTURES _____ I am pleased with the color and looks of the denture and am ready to have them processed. I also realize that adjustments will need to be made after delivery of my new denture.

        SignatureX_ _Dan Smith_____ Date _3-4-97_

ORTHO _____ I understand that _____ is in need of an orthodontic consultation and that if I delay in getting treatment done, that (his/her/my) condition could worsen or be harder to treat later in life, or no longer be treatable without surgery.

        Signature _____ Date _____

X-RAYS _____ I _____, understand that without dental x-rays, Hartland Dental Group is unable to diagnose many conditions that may exist and can only be seen on x-ray; including, but not limited to: cavities, faulty overhanging fillings, abcesses, and other bony defects.

        Signature _____ Date _____

Figure 3-28. Patient consent form.

In general practice, it is often necessary to refer patients to a dental specialist. In such cases, the referral form becomes a written communication between the referring doctor and the dental specialist. It is important to be as specific as possible in the request for evaluation and treatment, and the form should be reviewed and explained to the patient by the doctor. The following figures are examples of commonly requested procedures (Figs. 3-29 to 3-32).

Figure 3-29. Referral form for a periodontist. Reproduced courtesy of Wayne D. Du Pont, DDS, PS, Auburn, Washington.

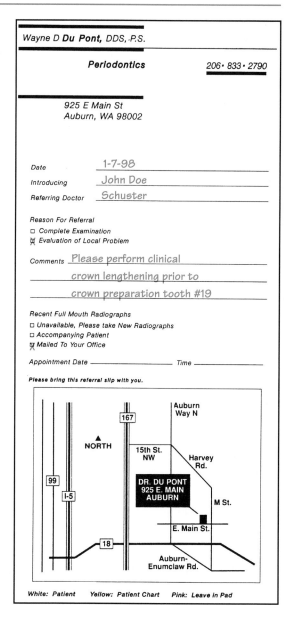

Wayne D **Du Pont,** DDS, P.S.

Periodontics   206 · 833 · 2790

925 E Main St
Auburn, WA 98002

Date   1-7-98

Introducing   John Doe

Referring Doctor   Schuster

Reason For Referral
☐ Complete Examination
☒ Evaluation of Local Problem

Comments   Please perform clinical
           crown lengthening prior to
           crown preparation tooth #19

Recent Full Mouth Radiographs
☐ Unavailable, Please take New Radiographs
☐ Accompanying Patient
☒ Mailed To Your Office

Appointment Date _____ Time _____

Please bring this referral slip with you.

White: Patient   Yellow: Patient Chart   Pink: Leave in Pad

JOHN DAVID WEST
D.D.S., M.S.D., P.S.

endodontics

American Association
of Endodontists
• **Specialist Member**

Date 1-8-98

Introducing __John Doe__

Referred by Dr. _Schuster_

Dr. Phone # _863-8138_ Receptionist _Layne_

Tooth or teeth to be treated _#19_

Requested completion date _2-8-98_

Comments:

    Please begin RCT #19

        Thanks!

Tacoma Mall Office Building
4301 S. Pine St., Suite 21
Tacoma, WA 98409-7293
Telephone: (206) 473-0101
1-800-424-ROOT
Fax: 206 473-6328

Please check appropriate needs

☒ Nonsurgical endodontic treatment
☐ Surgical endodontic treatment
☐ Retreatment
☐ Post and core
☒ Post space
☐ Diagnosis
☐ Apexification
☐ Gingivo and/or Osteoplasty
   (increase crown length)
☐ Post removal
☐ Perforation repair
☐ Pulpless bleaching
☐ Other service

Please send in advance of patient

Figure 3-30. Referral form for an endodontist. Reproduced courtesy of John David West,
DDS, MSD, PS, Tacoma, Washington.

Figure 3-31. Referral form for an
orthodontist. Reproduced courtesy
of David L. Crouch, DDS, MSD, Puyallup, Washington.

David L. Crouch, DDS, MSD
Orthodontics for Children,
Adolescents, and Adults

Woodcreek Office Park
1706 Meridian South, Suite 110
Puyallup, Washington 98371
(206) 848-9591

Date __1-8-98__

Introducing: __John Doe__

Referred by: __Schuster__

Comments: __Please eval. #19__
__for molar uprighting.__

Thanks!

INITIAL EXAMINATION

At the preliminary orthodontic evaluation one can
expect to discuss:

• THE GENERAL ORTHODONTIC
CONDITION

• IF TREATMENT IS NEEDED AND OPTIONS

• ESTIMATED LENGTH OF CARE

• APPROXIMATE FEES

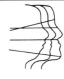

Ronald H. McCombs, D.D.S., M.S.
and Associates
Practice Limited To Oral and Maxillofacial Surgery

Member
American Association of
Oral and Maxillofacial Surgeons

10217 125th St., Ct., E., #300
Puyallup, WA 98374
(206) 770-1000

Introducing:

    John Doe
_____

Referred by Doctor:

    Schuster _____ Date: *1-8-98* _____

INSTRUCTIONS TO PATIENT

1. Please call 770-1000, for consultation appointment.

2. Minors (anyone under the age of 18) must be accompanied by parents or legal guardian at the time of examination.

3. If you have recent x-rays of the surgical area, please bring them with you, or ask your dentist to foreward them to our office.

4. No food, water, or liquids should be taken for 8 (eight) hours before your surgery appointment if a general anesthetic is to be used. General anesthetic patients must be accompanied by a responsible adult.

5. A consultation appointment is usually necessary to determine the extent of surgery, and the type of anesthesia, in simple procedures such as one or two uncomplicated extractions without general anesthesia, no examination appointment is usually necessary.

6. Estimates or surgical fees given only after consultation.

7. All fees are payable at time of surgery unless financial arrangements are made in advance.

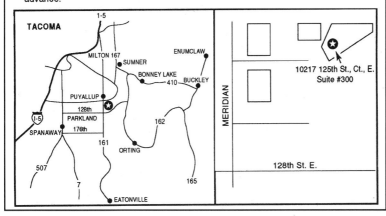

Figure 3-32. Referral form for an oral surgeon. Reproduced courtesy of Ronald H. McCombs, DDS, MS, Puyallup, Washington.

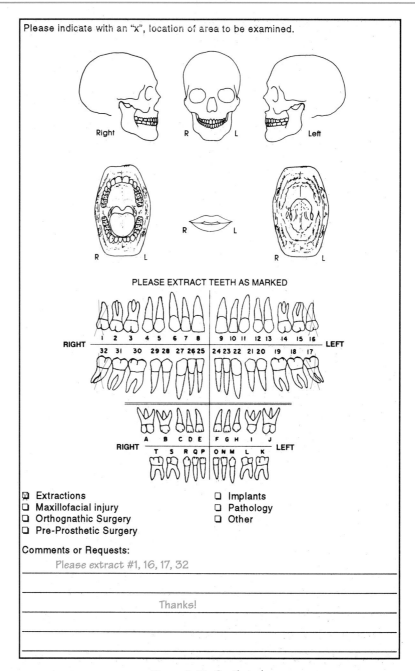

Please indicate with an "x", location of area to be examined.

Right   R   L   Left

PLEASE EXTRACT TEETH AS MARKED

RIGHT   1 2 3 4 5 6 7 8   9 10 11 12 13 14 15 16   LEFT
32 31 30 29 28 27 26 25   24 23 22 21 20 19 18 17

RIGHT   A B C D E   F G H I J   LEFT
T S R Q P   O N M L K

❑ Extractions   ❑ Implants
❑ Maxillofacial injury   ❑ Pathology
❑ Orthognathic Surgery   ❑ Other
❑ Pre-Prosthetic Surgery

Comments or Requests:
   Please extract #1, 16, 17, 32

                    Thanks!

Figure 3-32. Continued

Study Questions

1. The medical history form "Notes" section must be _____ and _____ each time the health history is reviewed.

2. Existing restorations are charted in _____ and recorded on the _____ form.

3. Teeth numbers and surfaces to be restored are charted in what color, recorded how, and on which form?

4. Every chart entry must end with what two items?

5. _____ is a commonly used broad-spectrum antibiotic with the following dose: _____.

6. A commonly used antibiotic for a penicillin-allergic patient is _____.

7. In the event of a medical emergency, the patient should be placed in what position?

8. After the patient has been placed in this position, what should be done next?

Clinical Procedures/ Behavioral Objectives and Rationale

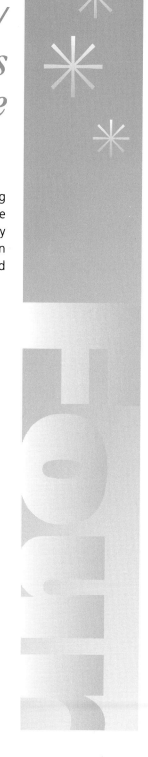

Objectives

When the dental assistant has mastered the material in Chapters 1–3, the following material can be studied. It is helpful for the dental assistant to be knowledgeable about the various clinical procedures in order to excel at the chairside and, as familiarity with the operations increases, to learn to anticipate the doctor's next move and begin interactive assisting. The material in this chapter provides behavioral objectives and rationales for the following clinical procedures:

Amalgam Procedure

Composite Procedure

Crown and Bridge Procedure

Root Canal Therapy

Removable Partial and Complete
    Dentures

Periodontal Therapy/Curettage
    and Scaling

Oral Surgery/Extractions

Amalgam Procedure

Behavioral Objectives	Rationale
1. Placement of dental dam	Isolates field; enhances vision; improves access; protects tongue, throat, and tissues; safeguards against swallowing unwanted materials
2. Preparation of tooth (G.V. Black's seven steps of cavity preparation)	1. Outline—creates border of restoration 2. Resistance—prevents displacement or fracture of enamel or dentin 3. Retention—prevents dislodgment of restoration 4. Convenience—gains access for insertion and finishing 5. Caries removal—eliminates disease 6. Finish—beveling or smoothing of the enamel walls of the preparation 7. Toilet—cavity debridement
3. Preparation of tooth (liner, base)	Liner or base covers or protects pulp from thermal stimuli and seals dentinal tubules
4. Placement of matrix and wedges	Confines alloy to preparation during condensation and approximates original tooth contours
5. Carving alloy	Restores anatomical contours and occlusion
6. Polishing alloy	Smoothes alloy surface, which decreases the available surface area for plaque adhesion and improves marginal adaptation

Composite Procedure

Behavioral Objectives	Rationale
1. Placement of dental dam	Isolates field; enhances vision; improves access; protects tongue, throat, and tissues; safeguards against swallowing unwanted materials
2. Preparation of tooth	G.V. Black's seven steps of cavity preparation (see "Amalgam Procedure")
3. Preparation of tooth (liner, base)	Liner or base covers or protects pulp from thermal stimuli and seals dentinal tubules
4. Acid etching of enamel	Provides mechanical retention for composite
5. Application of primer, bonding resin, and composite resin	Mechanically bonds to dentin and enamel
6. Polishing composite	Smoothes composite surface, which improves esthetics and marginal adaptation

Crown and Bridge Procedure

Behavioral Objectives	Rationale
1. Preparation of tooth	Caries removal and retention for restoration, draw, path of insertion
2. Use of wax tab	Check for occlusal clearance
3. Taking bite registration	Use to mount upper and lower models on articulator
4. Placing retraction cord	Temporarily deflects tissue for impression; protects gingival sulcus and epithelial attachment
5. Fabrication of temporary crown	Maintains mesial-distal tooth position in arch; maintains occlusion; reduces tooth sensitivity
6. Evaluation of the casting	
a. Aerosol spray (Occlude or Fit-Checker)	Check for internal interference
b. Floss	Check proximal contacts
c. Mylar/articulating paper	Check occlusion
7. Cementation	Causes casting to adhere to tooth
8. Cleanup	Check sulcus and remove excess cement

Root Canal Therapy

Behavioral Objectives	Rationale
1. Open and broach procedure	Relieves internal pressure and provides channel for drainage
2. Instrumentation	Removes infected material and provides access for obturation
3. Irrigation (root canal preparation and sodium hypochlorite)	Emulsifies pulp tissue and lubricates root canal system
4. Obturation	Seals tooth from oral cavity and surrounding periapical tissues

Behavioral Objectives	Rationale
1. Final impressions	Accurately reproduce teeth, tissue, and anatomical landmarks necessary for retention, resistance, and stability of prosthesis
2. Removable partial denture framework try-in	Evaluate and adjust fit of clasps before acrylic processing
3. Complete denture maxillary–mandibular relations	Evaluate vertical dimension, closest speaking space, lip support, overjet, midline, smile line
4. Complete denture clinical try-in	Reevaluate criteria and esthetics for complete denture maxillary–mandibular relations before processing
5. Delivery	Replace missing teeth and prevent collapse of remaining teeth and facial structures

Periodontal Therapy/Curettage and Scaling

Behavioral Objectives	Rationale
1. Curettage, scaling, and root planning	Subgingival plaque becomes subgingival calculus, which is sharp and irritating to the gums. Irritated gums turn red, swell, and become infected (gingivitis). If the gums remain infected, the bone becomes infected, resulting in bone loss (periodontal disease). Calculus must be removed by mechanical devices in the dental office.
2. Coronal polish	Supragingival polishing creates a smooth surface *following* scaling, thus decreasing the opportunity for plaque adhesion. It should not serve as a substitute for scaling.

Behavioral Objectives	Rationale
1. Use of surgical curette	Severs epithelial attachment
2. Use of elevators	Expands bony socket; provides apical pressure, forcing root(s) coronally
3. Use of forceps	Further expands bony socket; delivers tooth by providing apical pressure, forcing tooth coronally

Study Questions

1. List five reasons for placement of the dental dam during restorative procedures.

2. What is the fifth step in G.V. Black's steps for cavity preparation?

3. Two important reasons for polishing amalgam are _____ and

   _____.

4. What are two results of properly placed retraction cord?

5. The goals of root canal instrumentation are _____ and

   _____.

6. Calculus can be removed by standard tooth-brushing techniques. T or F

7. Use of the surgical curette during a tooth extraction serves what important function?

Appendix A:
Answers to Study Questions

Chapter 1

1. What four items are common to every tray setup? *AIR-WATER TIP, HVE, COTTON ROLLS, 2×2s*
2. What is the first thing that is discussed with the patient and recorded in the chart after the patient has been seated? *HEALTH HISTORY*
3. What is the first thing that is done after the doctor has entered the operatory during a new patient examination appointment? *DOCTOR IS INTRODUCED TO PATIENT*
4. Existing restorations are charted in *BLUE* and recorded on the *INITIAL CLINICAL EXAMINATION FORM.*
5. Tooth surfaces to be restored are charted in *RED* and listed in the order to be treated on the *TREATMENT PLAN FORM.*
6. What question do you ask the doctor before releasing the patient? *WHAT IS THE NEXT APPOINTMENT?*
7. An appropriate bur for the high-speed handpiece to begin an amalgam procedure is *56,* for the slow-speed handpiece *6.*
8. Appropriate burs for the high-speed handpiece to begin a composite procedure are *330* or *56.*
9. A dental dam is (optional or *MANDATORY*) for a root canal procedure.
10. A dental dam is prepared with *ONE* hole(s) for a root canal procedure.
11. *ORTHODONTIC THREE-PRONG* pliers are used to adjust the removable partial denture framework.
12. The dental assistant explains and has the oral surgery patient sign the *CONSENT FORM* prior to the procedure and explains the *POSTOPERATIVE* instructions to the patient following the procedure.
13. Maxillary universal forceps are *#150,* while mandibular universal forceps are *#151.*

Chapter 2

1. Topical anesthetic for an inferior alveolar nerve block is placed between the *PTERYGO-MANDIBULAR RAPHE* and the *CORONOID NOTCH* approximately *ONE* cm above the occlusal plane.
2. Topical anesthetic should be held in place for *1–2* minutes.
3. Dental dam septa can be inverted using *AIR* and a *BLUNT ENDED INSTRUMENT.*
4. A dental dam prepared for an endodontic procedure should have how many holes? *ONE*

5. When placing the HVE, the tip should be *PARALLEL* to the buccal or lingual surface of the tooth.

6. The *REVERSE PALM-THUMB* grasp is the preferred hand position for the HVE because more *CONTROL* is gained.

7. When passing instruments during a procedure, the dental assistant receives the used instrument with which finger? *LITTLE*

8. After receiving the used instrument, the dental assistant passes the new instrument with the nib *UP* when working on maxillary teeth and *DOWN* when working on mandibular teeth.

9. When taking radiographs, the white side of the film packet should be facing the x-ray tube. *T*

10. When taking bitewing or periapical radiographs, the film should be placed (buccal or *LINGUAL*) to the teeth.

11. When placing the Tofflemire matrix and retainer, the retainer must always rest against the *BUCCAL* surfaces of the teeth.

12. The opening of the slot on the Tofflemire retainer must always point toward the *GIN-GIVA* in order to facilitate removal.

13. When preparing the daysheet, each tooth to be restored has its own line with what three pieces of information? *TOOTH #, SURFACES TO BE RESTORED, RESTORATIVE MATERIAL*

Chapter 3

1. The medical history form "Notes" section must be *DATED* and *SIGNED* each time the health history is reviewed.

2. Existing restorations are charted in *BLUE* and recorded on the *INITIAL CLINICAL EXAMINATION* form.

3. Teeth number and surfaces to be restored are charted in what color, recorded how, and on which form? *RED, IN THE ORDER TO BE TREATED, TREATMENT PLAN FORM*

4. Every chart entry must end with what two items? *NEXT APPOINTMENT (N.A.), INITIALS*

5. *AMOXICILLIN* is a commonly used broad-spectrum antibiotic with the following dose: *500mg, 29 tabs, 2stat then q6h until gone.*

6. A commonly used antibiotic for a penicillin-allergic patient is *ERYTHROMYCIN*.

7. In the event of a medical emergency, the patient should be placed in what position? *SUPINE*

8. After the patient has been placed in the above position, what should be done next? *AIRWAY CLEARED*

Chapter 4

1. List five reasons for placement of the dental dam during restorative procedures. *ISOLATION OF FIELD; ENHANCED VISION; IMPROVED ACCESS; PROTECTS TONGUE, THROAT, AND TISSUES; SAFEGUARDS AGAINST SWALLOWING UNWANTED MATERIALS*

2. What is the fifth step in G.V. Black's steps for cavity preparation? *CARIES REMOVAL*
3. Two important reasons for polishing amalgam are *DECREASES PLAQUE RETENTION* and *INCREASES MARGINAL ADAPTATION.*
4. What are two results of properly placed retraction cord? *TEMPORARILY DEFLECTS GINGIVAL TISSUE FOR IMPRESSION and PROTECTS GINGIVAL SULCUS AND EPITHELIAL ATTACHMENT.*
5. The goals of root canal instrumentation are *TO REMOVE INFECTED MATERIAL* and *TO PROVIDE ACCESS FOR OBTURATION.*
6. Calculus can be removed by standard tooth-brushing techniques. *F*
7. Use of the surgical curette during a tooth extraction serves what important function? *SEVERS EPITHELIAL ATTACHMENT*

Appendix B:
Commonly Used Abbreviations

A	amalgam	I	incisal
adj	adjust	IA	inferior alveolar nerve
ASA	anterior superior alveolar nerve	Imp	impression
B	buccal	Inf	infiltrate
BU	crown buildup	L	lingual
BWX	bitewing radiographs	LA	lower anterior
C	composite	LB	long buccal nerve
CC	chief concern	Lido	lidocaine
CD	complete denture	LL	lower left
Calc	calculus	LR	lower right
Carbo	3% carbocaine	M	mesial
Cem	cement	Mod	moderate
Citn	4% citanest	NG	nightguard
CMCP	camphorated paramonochlorophenol	NP	new patient
Cp	cotton pellet	O	occlusal
D	distal	O&B	open and broach
EDTA	ethylenediaminetetraacetic acid	OHI	oral hygiene instruction
EES	erythromycin ethylsuccinate	PAN	panorex radiograph
E-mycin	erythromycin stearate	PAX	periapical radiograph
Epi	epinephrine	Pen VK	penicillin VK
F	facial	PFC	porcelain fused to metal crown
FGC	full gold crown	PIP	pressure indicator paste
FMX	full mouth series of radiographs	PSA	posterior superior alveolar nerve
Fl	fluoride	Pt	patient
Gp	gutta percha	RCT	root canal therapy
Hx	history	Rec	recommended
		Reg	registration

RPD	removable partial denture	UA	upper anterior
Rx	prescription	UL	upper left
Sub	subgingival	UR	upper right
Supra	supragingival	VDO	vertical dimension of occlusion
Tb	toothbrush	VDR	vertical dimension at rest
TE	tooth extraction	W/	with
Temp	temporary	WL	working length
Tx	treatment	WNL	within normal limits

Appendix C:
Student Evaluation Sheets

The following student evaluation sheets are intended to provide the dental assistant with written feedback on a daily basis for various duties and clinical procedures. The evaluations are based on typical duties required in a three-operatory dental clinic, including office administration and infection control.

Evaluation: Operatory Procedures (OP-1 and OP-2)

Student _____

Date _____ Instructor's initials _____

Scoring Criteria:

Acceptable   (3)—Ideal/Excellent/Perfect

                    (2)—Minor deviations from ideal

Unacceptable   (1)—Correctable deviations; corrections necessary to avoid significant
                    compromise

                    (0)—Major deviations; uncorrectable; may indicate lack of skill and/or concept

Category	Score
Operatory organized and clean	_____
Patient and light properly positioned	_____
Handpieces/tray preparation complete	_____
Anesthetic preparation and transfer	_____
Proper isolation/dental dam application	_____
Oral evacuation technique	_____
Rinse and dry technique	_____
Proper instrument transfer	_____
Mixes and delivers materials/takes accurate alginate impressions	_____
Coronal polish technique and oral hygiene instruction	_____
Updates medical history/makes accurate chart entries	_____
Completed treatment marked off on Treatment Plan form	_____
Demonstrates knowledge of materials and procedures	_____
Professional conduct	_____

Total Points Possible = 42   **Total Points = _____**

Evaluation: Operatory Procedures (OP-3)

Student _____

Date _____ Instructor's initials _____

Scoring Criteria:

Acceptable   (3)—Ideal/Excellent/Perfect
                   (2)—Minor deviations from ideal
Unacceptable   (1)—Correctable deviations; corrections necessary to avoid significant
                   compromise
                   (0)—Major deviations; uncorrectable; may indicate lack of skill and/or concept

Category	Score
Operatory organized and clean	_____
Patient and light properly positioned	_____
Handpieces/tray preparation complete	_____
Proper instrument transfer	_____
Takes accurate alginate impressions	_____
Coronal polish technique and oral hygiene instruction	_____
Correctly takes, processes, and mounts dental radiographs	_____
Obtains accurate panoramic radiograph	_____
Demonstrates knowledge of radiology and equipment	_____
Updates medical history/makes accurate chart entries	_____
Correctly charts existing restorations on Initial Clinical Examination form	_____
Prepares treatment plan in sequence after review with the doctor	_____
Correctly follows appropriate handbook procedures	_____
Professional conduct	_____

Total Points Possible = 42   **Total Points = _____**

Evaluation: Dental Office Administration

Student _____

Date _____ Instructor's initials _____

Scoring Criteria:

Acceptable   (3)—Ideal/Excellent/Perfect
                    (2)—Minor deviations from ideal
Unacceptable   (1)—Correctable deviations; corrections necessary to avoid significant
                    compromise
                    (0)—Major deviations; uncorrectable; may indicate lack of skill and/or concept

Category	Score
Updates Daysheets (hall, lab, OP-1, OP-2, OP-3)	_____
Correctly takes/relays messages to the doctor	_____
Correctly prepares patient dental charts	_____
Identifies Medical History form risk factors	_____
Explains fees, dental programs, and procedures	_____
Correctly coordinates patients with available operatories	_____
Develops and maintains patient appointment book	_____
Correctly follows appropriate handbook procedures	_____
Lists day-end production total on Daysheet	_____
Correctly prepares next-day Daysheet	_____
Leaves desk area clean and organized	_____

Total Points Possible = 33   **Total Points = _____**

Evaluation: Infection Control/Sterilization

Student _____

Date _____ Instructor's initials _____

Scoring Criteria:

Acceptable	(3)—Ideal/Excellent/Perfect
	(2)—Minor deviations from ideal
Unacceptable	(1)—Correctable deviations; corrections necessary to avoid significant compromise
	(0)—Major deviations; uncorrectable; may indicate lack of skill and/or concept

Category	Score
Follows appropriate OSHA/state regulations and guidelines	_____
Correctly handles/identifies hazardous materials	_____
Disinfects/sterilizes dental instruments, handpieces, and trays	_____
Effectively acts as backup/helper to chairside assistants	_____
Properly prepares tray setups	_____

Total Points Possible = 15   **Total Points = _____**

References

Black, G.V.: *Operative Dentistry,* vols. I–IV. Chicago, Medico-Dental Publishing Co., 1908.

Craig, R.G.: *Restorative Dentistry Materials,* 9th ed. St. Louis, C.V. Mosby Co., 1993.

Ehrlich, A., and Torres, H.O.: *Essentials of Dental Assisting,* 2nd ed. Philadelphia, W.B. Saunders Co., 1996.

Infection Control Recommendations for the Dental Office and the Dental Laboratory. Chicago, American Dental Association, August 1992.

Intraoral Radiography with Rinn XCP/BAI Instruments. Elgin, IL, Rinn Corp., 1993.

Malamed, S.F., and Sheppard, G.A.: *Handbook of Emergencies in the Dental Office,* 3rd ed. St. Louis, C.V. Mosby Co., 1987.

Sturdevant, C.M., Barton, R.E., Sockwell, C.L., and Strickland, W.D.: *The Art and Science of Operative Dentistry,* 2nd ed. St. Louis, C.V. Mosby Co., 1985.

Torres, H.O., and Ehrlich, A.: *Modern Dental Assisting,* 5th ed. Philadelphia, W.B. Saunders Co., 1995.

Index

Note: Page numbers in *italics* refer to illustrations.